WEIGHT LOSS PSYCHOLOGY FOR WOMEN SERIES

Part One

and

I0424779

Part Two

FELICIA URBAN RN, MSN

Interested in more content by
<u>Felicia Urban</u>?

Come visit us on the Weight Loss Psychology Series <u>website</u> and don't forget to hit that <u>subscribe button</u> to stay up to date on all new content! https://geni.us/WLPSeries

Interact with Weight Loss Psychology community by joining the <u>Facebook page</u>

Interact with Weight Loss Psychology community by joining the <u>Facebook group</u>

Interested in the author and her other books? Take a look on <u>Amazon</u>

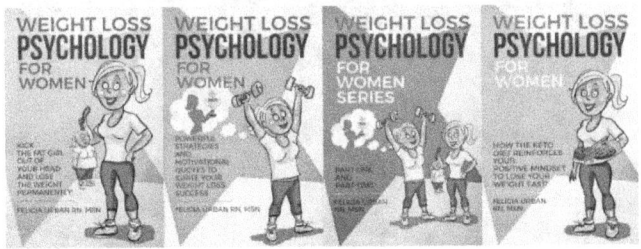

Felica Urban RN, MSN

About the author

The author, Felicia Urban RN, MSN, suffered from weight loss and gain until she was thirty years old. At age 29, she was at her highest weight ever of 234 pounds.

She lost an amazing 90 pounds over the course of one year! She earnestly sought to understand what made her weight loss journey so difficult in the past and how to recapture and maintain her successful mindset that lead to her astounding 90-pound weight loss.

Her search led her to land a job at a popular weight loss physician's clinic. Here she interviewed and obtained the weight loss history of an estimated 500 plus patients who were all struggling to win the battle of permanent weight loss. One thing became clear to Ms. Urban, mindset prepping and maintenance of that mindset are essential to permanent weight loss success!

Most diets will work if followed closely. The difference between success and failure, Ms. Urban found, wasn't the diet plan, it was the proper mindset! Upon learning this, Ms. Urban has made it her life's mission to teach as many people as she can how to achieve proper mindset and reach their goals as she has done herself.

Ms. Urban lives on the outskirts of Orlando, Florida with her husband, three kids, four horses, three dogs and one cat named, "Frodo". She loves paintball, camping and growing organic vegetables. She now has a successful private practice as a weight-loss and life coach.

Table of Contents

KICK THE FAT GIRL OUT OF YOUR HEAD AND LOSE WEIGHT!

INTRODUCTION 1

The Tools Needed 2

Take Your Time 3

CHAPTER 1 – LOOKING INWARD 4

Identifying Trauma 4

Confront the Root Issue 5

Why do I Eat? 6

Finding a New Goal 7

Other Benefits 9

Avoid Triggers 10

Avoiding Punishment 10

Small Wins and Losses 12

Positive Reinforcement 13

CHAPTER 2 - RECENT MINDSET RESEARCH 14

You Are Not Alone 15

How Being Overweight Affects Your Mind 17

The Effects on the Hippocampus 19

Sneaky Addictive Foods 20

How You Were Raised Counts 23

Pregnant Moms Who Exercise Will Likely Give Birth to Healthy Kids 26

Mindfulness Training Helps 28

Portion Control 30

CHAPTER 3 – STRATEGIES AND MIND EXERCISES 35

Keep a Journal 35

Avoid the Scale 36

The Calorie Myth 36

Talk About It 37

Affirmations 38

CHAPTER 4 – TIME MANAGEMENT 40

Practice Patience 40

There is No Rush 41

Set Small Goals 41

Don't Wait for Monday 42

Something to Tend 43

Lifestyle Change 43

Keeping the Weight Off 44

Change Things Up 45

Don't Revel in Regret 46

It Gets Easier 46

CONCLUSION 48

Weight-Loss Mindset Review 48

Be Proud of Yourself 49

Remember, it is Up to You 49

POWERFUL STRATEGIES AND MOTIVATIONAL QUOTES TO IGNITE YOUR WEIGHT LOSS SUCCESS!

INTRODUCTION 51

CHAPTER 1 – ENHANCE YOUR MOTIVATION 56

Your Dream Outfit 60

Studies on Habit.. 63

Research on Motivation....................................... 65

Your Reason for Motivation............................... 67

CHAPTER 2 – NEVER GIVE UP! 70

Stay the Course 73

Starting Over is Harder Than Picking It Back Up 76

The Journey is Worth it in the End! 79

Journaling 82

Triggers 84

CHAPTER 3 – BEING ON TOP OF YOUR GAME 87

Saying No 90

Comparing Yourself 94

Planning Ahead 97

Moments of Stress 102

Travel 104

Be Prepared When You Forget 107

Going to Restaurants 108

Parties 110

Your Hormones 112

Weighing Yourself 113

CHAPTER 4 – GET BACK UP! 116

How You are Reacting 118

Speak to Yourself Like You Would a Friend ... 121

Have a Mess Up Strategy 123

Never Make Yourself Feel Guilty...................... 125

CHAPTER 5 – A LIFELONG JOURNEY 127

Finding Support Groups.................................... 129

Start Your Own Group...................................... 131

Setting Goals 132

Rewards Over Punishments 134

Give Yourself Permission 135

Always Look to the Root................................... 137

Binge Eating... 138

CHAPTER 6 – POSITIVE RELATIONSHIPS
.... 140

How You Were Raised Counts.......................... 143

Those That Bring You Down............................. 145

Don't Be Self-Conscious at the Gym 148

CHAPTER 7 - AN INDIVIDUAL'S WORTH. 150

Weight Loss Affirmations................................. 152

Write to Yourself When in a Good Mood 155

Mental Fitness 156

Rework Your Relationship with Food 157

Start Cooking 159

CHAPTER 8 - LIVE IN GRATITUDE 161

Help Others Achieve What You Have Achieved
.... 162

Having Fun with Exercise 162

Diet Mentality 163

CONCLUSION 165

REFERENCES 168

WEIGHT LOSS PSYCHOLOGY FOR WOMEN

Kick the Fat Girl Out of Your Head and Lose Weight!

FELICIA URBAN RN, MSN

Introduction

Some diets allow you to eat anything you want, as long as you do so within a few hours in the day. Other diets allow you to eat cookies, but the truth is, those cookies taste like cardboard. There are so many tricks, hacks, and crazy regimens one can use to try and lose weight. The reality is, if the mindset is not there to lose weight, it is not going to happen.

Finding diets, learning about different foods, and understanding how weight loss occurs are all simple things that anyone can achieve. When it comes time to actually start losing the weight, however, that is when a lot of people drop out. The reason why so many people fail to keep up with their diets is not because of what foods they are choosing to eat or which spin class they are enrolled in. It is because their minds have not caught up to what their hearts actually want.

There is a root issue for why someone can't lose weight. Food for some people becomes a comfort that not everyone is ready to let go of. Whether someone hates eating veggies and only eats junk, or if someone binges healthy food, there is a reason why we all have our certain eating habits. By digging deep into our past, present, and goals for the future, we can discover that the key to losing weight is not in a pill or program. It is all in our head.

The Tools Needed

If you walk into any given store at any point the week after New Year's Day, there will likely be displays and areas filled with weight-loss gear, workout clothes, and everything you need to lose weight. There is this illusion that if you buy a bunch of workout stuff, the motivation to actually workout will follow. This method can work for some people, but for the most part, there are not exact tools needed to lose weight. You might use resistance bands, weighted ankle straps, and the cutest matching sports bra and leggings set, but the weight is not going to come off unless you have reached the right mindset.

The only tool necessary to lose weight is your brain. You can find ways to work out without any gear or extra supplements. These certainly help make things easier, and many people find help from having different tools of motivation. The key—the most important tool of all—is a mindset that is ready to confront the issues and work through them in order to achieve weight-loss goals.

Having a clear goal as well as a plan of attack are the next two important tools needed to make sure that you are going to be able to lose the weight once and for all, as well as the tools needed to make sure the weight does not come back.

Take Your Time

Weight loss is a journey, not just a weekend trip. That being said, it is going to take some time to actually achieve your goals. You likely won't find it to be an easy, casual journey either. You are going to run into some bumps and slipups that might make it hard to recover. There are going to be moments when you ask if it is worth it all in the end and other times where you question why you are even doing what you are. It is not going to be an easy or quick thing. If it were, you would have done it by now.

All of this is important to accept when beginning a weight-loss regimen. Accept the fact that there is no small fix for weight loss. There are pills you can take that help a bit, and other supplements that might help you lose some pounds. To really change your life and finally become the person you have always wanted to be, however, it is going to take some time. Weight loss is a process that requires patience, acceptance, and dedication. Though it might be tough at first, it does get easier. Achieving your goals is ALWAYS worth it in the end.

Chapter 1 – Looking Inward

Sometimes, our weight-loss goals are all about just making sure that we look good in a bikini. Though we want our outsides to look good, we have to make sure the insides are looking even better. This does not mean your bones and blood, but your heart and mind. Is your brain ready to go through such a journey? Is your heart really in it in the end?

If you want to make sure you look good, you can't expect to do so while completely disregarding the inner workings of all the other systems in your body. This journey should be a healthy one, and that does not mean just looking the part. Crash dieting, binging and purging, and using extreme weight-loss supplements are all just attempts at fixing something that weight loss will not cure.

What's more important than just making sure you can fit into the right-sized outfit for an upcoming wedding is making sure that your mental state is strong enough to handle it if you don't end up fitting. The first step in doing this is making sure that you look at the root issue rather than looking at what you see in the mirror.

Identifying Trauma

Losing weight means looking at our past lives to determine what might have caused our current bad behaviors. Sometimes, this means having to look at a specific childhood trauma. Trauma can be defined as any sort of disturbing, unsettling, or distressing occurrence. Sometimes, this one small instance sticks with us forever, such as a car accident or natural disaster. Other times, trauma presents itself in other forms such as having an abusive or alcoholic parent.

You might already realize your traumas, or maybe it will take some time to understand the things you endured as a child that still disturb you as an adult. In order to make sure that you can combat everything that might come your way as you work out, it is important to determine what trauma still follows you. Perhaps you eat when you feel stressed because, as a child, you would eat snacks in the kitchen while your parents fought in the other room. Maybe you can't go to the gym because it is located next to a dentist's office, and you had a traumatic teeth-cleaning experience as a child. Knowingly or not, your trauma is likely playing into your current eating and dieting habits.

Confront the Root Issue

The thing about most of our problems is that you can usually trace them back to one big issue. We're like trees. We have all these branches, leaves, and little inner workings that all lead back to the trunk. Without that big deep root, nothing else would exist. For the most part, we can trace our current issues back to one, or maybe two root issues.

For example, many control issues come from a place of fear of abandonment. Those that look for ways to take control of their lives, whether it is in work or social settings, usually can trace their issues back to a time when they felt like they had no control. Maybe a parent left, or they dealt with loss at a young age. This control might come into play in their eating habits as well. By identifying past traumas and looking inward, you will be surprised at how easily you can confront the root issue to most of your problems.

This is not always going to be the case with everything in life. Certain illnesses or money issues are things that might spring up later in life, and we can't always connect these issues to our childhoods. When it comes to eating, however, that is usually an emotional experience for someone, which means they can trace it to their past life and analyze how or why that specific eating habit was created.

Why do I Eat?

Before dieting, continue with your current eating habits. Take note while you are eating about how it makes you feel. If you are sitting on the couch and you decide to eat the entire bag of chips when it only takes a handful to feel full, make a note of why you decided to do that. You won't always be able to attack the root issue right away, but you might start determining why you feel the need to overeat when you know you shouldn't. Maybe you will realize you are only eating because you are bored, or perhaps it is just a habit of convenience. Maybe you realize that you don't even feel that good while eating the chips, but you do it anyway.

Always ask why whenever you are eating. Why am I choosing to eat this fast food when there is food in the fridge? Why am I eating two sandwiches when it only takes one? Why do I keep eating this dip even though I'm already full? The more you ask why and question the behaviors you are able to identify, the better you will be able to come up with a solution to confront and attack your root issues.

Finding a New Goal

What's your goal for losing weight? Is it to fit into a dress? Is it so you can get a new boyfriend/girlfriend? Is it so you have a flat stomach or so your face is not as round? If your goal for losing weight is just to look good, you should find a new goal. That is the reason many people want to lose weight in the first place. They just want to be "hot" or "sexy," with a fit body that attracts other people, or at least gets positive attention from those around them. It is not uncommon to have vanity goals when it comes to losing weight. It is also not uncommon for people to give up on their weight-loss goals.

Looking good should just be an added bonus for losing weight. If you don't find a substantial and deeply-rooted goal for losing weight, you won't be as likely to keep up with your hopes. Instead of losing weight just to be hot, you have to find a reason that is more important.

Lose weight because you want to have a healthy heart. Having a healthy heart means that you will live longer, which means you'll get to spend more time with your friends and family. When you create a goal that has more meaning, you will be able to stick to that goal more easily than if you just want to be able to slip into some skinny jeans.

Create smaller goals that are important as well. Lose the weight because you want to be able to walk up a flight of stairs without having to catch your breath. Lose weight because you want to make it easier to move when it comes time to switch apartments. Lose weight because you will have the assurance that you can outrun anyone in case of some sort of zombie apocalypse.

Just remember that looking the best out of everyone at your high school reunion will just be the added bonus to losing weight, not the overall goal. That way, you will be able to stick to your weight-loss regimen if you do hit a certain body weight.

It is also important to understand your current value and beauty. You are not ugly, unattractive, or undesirable at any weight. That beautiful person exists inside of you, and it will show through no matter what size you are. You just have to recognize that wonderful person and treat them well, not shame them for not looking "sexy" enough.

Other Benefits

When creating a goal, you have to look at the overall benefits that will come along with achieving certain milestones. By doing this, you will be able to fulfill your goals better because you have a clear map of what benefits you will be reaping.

There are so many benefits to losing weight besides just the way you might look. Losing weight could help someone manage with their anxiety and depression. Working out releases endorphins, and certain junk food has been linked to producing depressive feelings.

Being more in shape allows someone to do things that someone out of shape, can't. You can go for walks with friends and not have to worry about what games you might play that could involve physical activity.

Being an overweight teenager and young adult is challenging because, at that age, there is so much pressure to look good. However, being overweight and in your forties or older is so much worse, and not even for beauty reasons. As our bodies age, no matter how healthy they are, certain things just don't work the way they used to. Our backs, knees, and hips start to not work as well as they used to and being overweight just puts more pressure on all these parts of our bodies. The older you get, the harder being overweight is on your body. It is also harder to lose weight the older you get. Losing the weight now, no matter what age, is always a better option than waiting and losing the weight later.

Avoid Triggers

Once you start identifying your trauma, it is time to look at what triggers might cause you to keep slipping up on your goals. This might include a bakery that you have to pass on your way home from work. Maybe different parties you frequent have buffet-style snacks always readily available. When you can start to identify what triggers surround you that cause you to eat, you can do your best to avoid these triggers, or at least be ready when they come about.

This might also include certain behaviors, experiences, or even people that make you feel like you have to eat. Maybe whenever you get in a fight with your boyfriend/girlfriend, you cope by binging out on some ice cream. Perhaps you feel like you can't sit down to watch a movie without having a snack in your hand. There are many different triggers we have on an individual level, but the main idea is that they need to be identified so it is easier to either avoid or confront them.

Avoiding Punishment

The biggest mistake we make when starting any sort of diet or weight-loss regimen is that we punish ourselves along the way. Whether the punishment comes from us not starting at the right time, slipping up on a strict diet, or just being regretful for not starting sooner, most of us are way too hard on ourselves. We say things to ourselves that are crueler than our worst bullies could imagine.

When we punish ourselves, whether it is just saying mean things in our heads or actually self-harming, we're forcing ourselves to feel dangerous emotions that might cause us to eat. Maybe you are mad at yourself for eating the free donuts your coworker brought into work. As a punishment that day, you skip lunch. On a more extreme level, maybe you hate yourself so much for being overweight for a long time that you go as far as to physically self-harm yourself.

Punishment is necessary for training dogs or teaching kids certain lessons. We punish bullies, criminals, and other people that exhibit bad behavior. You don't need to punish yourself, however. You should be your own best friend, so instead of making yourself feel terrible for not reaching a goal, remind yourself that you need to take care of yourself because you deserve it.

We still have to stay strict with our goals, but positive reinforcement will always be better than tearing yourself apart. When you constantly belittle yourself, you are seeing yourself as someone that does not deserve happiness. You might be so hard on yourself that you get to a point where you question whether you even deserve to have a healthy body.

Go at your own pace and start dieting and exercising when you are ready. Right now, however, you have to make a promise to yourself that you are going to go a little easier on yourself. No more calling yourself dumb, lazy, or ugly. When you look in the mirror, remember to point out the things you like, reminding yourself of how much beauty you really do have to offer. It is an uncomfortable feeling for some, but it is incredibly important in order to make sure that you fulfill your weight-loss goals.

Small Wins and Losses

Having an overall goal is important, but make sure to set small goals in between. For example, maybe your overall goal is to lose fifty pounds in a year. A small goal, then, would be to lose five pounds. Instead of waiting to celebrate until you lose the big fifty, have five- or ten-pound milestones. Celebrate that you are doing it! Just knowing you need to start living healthier is a huge thing, as not many people are willing to admit to themselves that they need to lose some weight and eat healthier. Once you actually start doing it, that is even more amazing! You should be incredibly proud, and the continual encouragement will only help you achieve your goals much easier in the end.

If you do slip up and do something that goes against your diet and exercise plan, just look at it as a small loss and not a complete failure. By reminding ourselves that we just made a small mistake, we can find the courage to keep going. When we tell ourselves we failed and have to start over, it can be hard to get back on track. Accept that you are going to have small losses along the way and remember that you will have just as many small victories.

Positive Reinforcement

Some instances require tough love, but that is not always going to work when it comes to losing weight. There are some people that are really hard on themselves, and it works to stick to a diet and exercise plan, but they might not be happy overall. The way to actually have a healthy body and a happy mind is to use positive reinforcement on yourself.

We get enough heat from the world we live in as it is. Our parents might be a source of "tough love," or maybe it is just the way that society makes some of us feel. Either way, we get enough of a feeling that we might not be "good enough" from other sources such that we don't need to do that to ourselves either. The key to having a consistent weight-loss mindset, geared towards achieving goals, is to use positive reinforcement.

Chapter 2 - Recent Mindset Research

Doing research is an important part of a weight-loss journey. Certain things might pose a health risk. If you try crash dieting, starvation periods, or other dangerous supplements, you might run the risk of doing more harm than good to your body. Before starting a serious weight-loss plan, it is always important to consult a physician. What might work for one person could be a dangerous risk for another. No two bodies are alike, so we can't always make assumptions about effects or results for different people participating in a weight-loss regimen.

What's more important is doing research on one's brain. Sometimes, that can be overlooked. When we lose weight, or at least when we start thinking of how we're going to cut the fat, we look at our stomachs and muscles, hoping to reduce the size of every physical element of our body. What's more important than improving on our muscles and other parts of our bodies is making sure that we're improving what's going on in our mind as well. It is easy to see that the way that we see food and ourselves is dependent on how our brain works. It goes much deeper than that, however.

There is an emphasis on mindset research, as it is clear that there is not yet a trick to losing weight. Instead of looking at how certain foods might affect our different body parts, we need to start looking at how food affects our mind. In addition to that, we need to look at our behavior, the choices we make, and the ways that we perceive different people and events in order to determine what the problem might be in our weight-loss journey. This emphasis also helps us to discover new ways to lose weight. It is not an answer of what our calorie count is, or how many minutes we clock at the gym. The key to achieving all of our weight-loss goals is hidden inside our brain, and scientists know this.

Being aware of the science behind a weight-loss mindset can help an individual be sure that they will actually find success with their plan. If we continue to ignore our brains and instead just workout our arms, abs, and legs, we'll never find easy success. It will always be about forcing ourselves to go to the gym, or moments of binging followed by punishment purging. By changing our mindset and the way we see food, as well as our perceptions of ourselves, we can make it easy to actually stick to a plan that helps us shed pounds and keep them off forever.

You Are Not Alone

Weight loss can be a lonely journey. It is up to us to get started, and we can only rely on ourselves to make sure that we follow through. It is likely that moments of loneliness are what led to our weight-loss struggles in the first place. Having to depend on just ourselves in this struggle can be what keeps us from achieving our goals. Sometimes, we are not strong enough to handle it all on our own, and that is okay. We need to remember that at first, we might need to ask for help. We shouldn't be expected to do it all by ourselves. When we become too dependent on ourselves for things that we can't always fix alone, there is a feeling of shame when we can't follow through.

When going through this journey, always remember that you are not alone. More than two in three adults are considered overweight. At this point, more people are struggling with their weight than those that are not. Even people that are not overweight still struggle with their perception of themselves as well as their overall body image. Don't be afraid to reach out and ask for help. Ask your parents for help in making sure they don't cook unhealthy meals or stock the fridge with junk food. Find a friend that also might be struggling with their weight and see if they want to start going on walks with you. The statistics prove that we are not in this alone, so there is no shame in reaching out for help.

One in thirteen adults have extreme obesity. When looking at weight-loss statistics like that, it is clear to see that you are certainly not alone in your weight-loss struggles. While these numbers might be concerning for our overall health and the way in which our society evaluates us, it can also be comforting to know that there are plenty people around us going through the same struggle. It is also a reminder that it is not our fault we got this way. We're certainly complicit in our own choices and can't blame the world for all of our health issues. It is a comforting reminder, however, to know that we're in a world set up for our weight issues. When a fast food meal is cheaper than a salad, we can't be so hard on ourselves when we do have moments of weakness.

How Being Overweight Affects Your Mind

Anyone can have a fit body, but that doesn't always mean they have a healthy mind. Mental illness like bipolar disorder, depression, and anxiety have the ability to affect many different people, no matter their size. With that in mind, it is also important to know that being overweight can have some seriously negative effects on your brain. Someone that struggles with mental illness and who is overweight might find that shedding some pounds actually improves their overall mental health as well.

Those who are overweight have issues with depression and anxiety more often than physically fit individuals. Part of this is because of the way society treats overweight individuals. When thin models are plastered all over billboards and other advertisements, it can be hard to not have a warped perception of bodies that don't look the same as those airbrushed beauties. However, more so than just the way our society affects body image, there are physical effects being overweight has on the brain.

Being overweight might lead to a higher risk of getting Alzheimer's or dementia. This is partially because excess weight affects the hippocampus, which we'll discuss in the next section. The foods that we eat, and how much oxygen we're giving our body, increase and decrease certain chemical levels in our brain which, in turn, may cause mental illnesses and disorders. These can end up leading to more weight loss on top of that as well.

There is a "dulling" effect on those who are overweight which leads to less enjoyment and pleasure from eating certain foods. When we drink sugary drinks all day, we become used to that constant sugar intake. This ends up warping our perception on sugary sweets, which means we get used to them and end up wanting more. In order to understand how this dulling effect works, start by giving up just one food you eat all the time. Before you start with a full-on diet, just give up something "bad for you" that you eat a few times a week, such as a sugary Starbucks drink, a nightly candy bar, a morning donut, or anything else that you consistently eat that is sweet. After just a week free of your item of choice, go ahead and indulge. You will be shocked at how sweet it might taste. This is because you have reduced your tolerance. You might find that the pleasure from just that one drink is so much greater than the consistent level of gratification you get from giving into your frequent indulgence.

The striatum is a part of our brain that is responsible for pleasure regulation. In overweight individuals, especially women, the striatum becomes weakened, giving us less pleasurable responses. This means that in terms of more than just food, we'll receive less pleasure from things that normally would bring us great joy. By eating healthier and exercising regularly, we're also taking care of our striatum which means our pleasure levels will rise back to where they should be. This is pleasure in all forms, whether it is from food, family, friends, music, sex, or anything else that brings us joy and happiness. The healthier our striatum, the more pleasure we'll feel.

The Effects on the Hippocampus

The hippocampus can actually grow with exercise. This part of your brain is responsible for the regulation of emotions. Those who struggle with their weight likely have some issues controlling their emotions, which will usually end up leading to more unhealthy eating patterns. When our emotions are out of whack, we make decisions we would not normally make with a clear head. This is when diets can really get messed up and lead to more weight gain and disappointment.

Those who are overweight have been known to have a lower ability to remember things, especially those aged eighteen to thirty-five. When our memory is warped, it can lead to plenty of other serious issues. We might forget how much we ate in a day, meaning we're not regulating our intake. We could also forget that we have not eaten, which is also a very unhealthy eating pattern. When we don't track how much we've been eating, it can end up causing cravings that can lead to sneaky weight gain.

Memory performance has been shown to improve in those that lose weight. Memory plays a role in weight management, as sometimes, our perspective on when to eat and when we last ate can be pretty hard to keep up with.

Post-traumatic stress and depression can cause damage to the hippocampus. Those that experience these mental illnesses, as well as individuals that are overweight, will only hurt their brain more, causing other dietary issues to arise. Our brains are precious organs that should be cared for meticulously. Luckily, our hippocampus can be improved if we work it out!

This is done through healthy diets that provide the brain with the nutrients it needs to function. Exercise is also an important part of working out your brain. Doing brain exercises, such as mindfulness strategies or games like Sudoku or word searches, will also improve cognitive function that will lead to other important health benefits other than just a reduction in weight.

Sneaky Addictive Foods

Losing weight sometimes has to be treated like an addiction. Those who are dependent on drugs, alcohol, sex, or other addictive substances share some qualities with individuals that might also be addicted to food. Someone that is addicted to alcohol first has to quit drinking, and then they can work on their mental health in order to make sure that they are keeping up with their sobriety. A person that is addicted to food can't just quit eating! There will always be temptations for an alcoholic in social settings, bars, and even the liquor section at grocery stores. Food is so much more present, however, and we have to eat it every single day of our lives, multiple times a day, in order to continue living!

The key to kicking a food addiction is to cut out the foods that you are addicted to. The habit of eating is an addiction in itself, and that is something different that needs to be confronted. However, there are certain foods that are physically addictive that can be very challenging for a person to give up. Avoiding these addictive foods is the key instead of just trying to moderate the amount. For any addictive food, it is important to look at what it can be replaced with.

The most addictive foods are filled with refined carbohydrates and added fat and sugar. This is because when those foods are eaten, there is a big increase of blood sugar which signals the pleasure centers of your brain, making you want even more. The reason why fast food is so good is because it is completely loaded with sugar. Even though Whoppers and Big Macs are not considered sweets, they still have a ton of added sugar that makes these foods addictive.

Tackling addiction is up to the individual. Some people are fine if they practice moderation. Other people can't even look at the food that they consider their addiction. In order to ensure that you don't fall back into a food addiction, it is important to figure out your plan for recovery. Are you going to be able to continue to surround yourself with the foods that tempt you on a daily basis? Or will you need to completely cut cupcakes out of your life? Sometimes, confronting addiction might also mean seeking professional help. There are psychologists that specialize in eating disorders who can provide extensive help to individuals with food addictions. There are also support groups filled with people that find themselves to be dependent upon or addicted to different foods and eating habits.

Chips and crackers are incredibly addicting for many reasons. They have added salt, which our bodies love, and they are not that filling on their own, meaning you will just keep loading up on them. Snacking is important to keep up our metabolism, but it needs to be extensively evaluated by the individual that is doing the snacking. Is it being done because you are actually hungry, or are you just bored? Maybe you are feeling anxious and need something to fill your hands, or perhaps you just looked at the snack and decided that it looked good.

Sweets like cake and ice cream are dangerous because of all the fat and sugar. If you are seriously addicted to sugar, you might also endure withdrawal symptoms when you don't get enough. Grumpiness, headaches, and other dangerous cravings are common symptoms of sugar addiction, so it is important that this individual issue is addressed in a weight-loss journey as well. You have to consider all of your dependencies and addictions in order to come up with a weight-loss plan that actually works.

How You Were Raised Counts

Those who have been overweight all their lives go through certain cycles. There is a period of unhealthy habits, the recognition that there needs to be a change, an attempt at change, the failure to follow through, and then back to a period of unhealthy habits. This cycle is present in many people that are overweight, but for those that were overweight kids and teens, it might be better understood. We might have also adopted this unhealthy cycle from our parents. Once we've found ourselves in this dangerous position, it can feel like clawing our way out when we actually decide we want to lose weight. If the pattern of behavior is not at first recognized, then we won't be able to determine the best method of breaking this unhealthy habit.

Studies have proven that kids who were weight-shamed go through cycles of binge eating and meal skipping that leads to self-loathing. A child that experiences criticism from their parents will start learning unhealthy methods of coping with weight and dieting. Eating is something that we've been doing all our lives, so the way that we eat now is certainly related to the way that we used to be taught to eat. Parents that might have body-shamed their kids by telling them they needed to lose weight or stop eating so much are responsible for causing self-loathing later in life.

Weight-shaming is not just blatantly telling someone that they are fat. It might also cloud diet encouragement. If your mom or dad always told you to try out a diet or suggested that you shouldn't eat a certain food, that was probably enough for you to feel a certain amount of shame about your weight. Even having a parent that continually talks about dieting is likely to make a child feel as though they should diet, too.

Many kids might grow up with moms who are constantly trying out new diets and fads. By seeing this is a kid, we end up going through the same phases. Maybe a parent was always saying things like, "I need to start my diet on Monday." This idea gets it in the kid's head that diets are something they should aim for, but only at a moment of convenience. The way a parent or even older sibling always talked about their body will play into how you might see your own body now. Perhaps your mom was always saying things like, "I hate my thighs; they are so big!" If a girl looks in the mirror and sees she has the same- shaped thighs as her mother, she'll end up thinking about how both she and her mother see those thighs as big, even though the mother never said anything directly to the girl about her body.

It is challenging because most parents just think they are helping. Parents that stock the fridge with Diet Coke instead of regular might think they are doing everyone a favor, when really, they are still supplying a form of addiction. Those that make sure to weigh their kids or track their workout routines could be doing so just because they want to make sure their kid is healthy, but they might not realize they are actually setting them up in a fearful manner in which dieting and exercising are an authoritative issue. Parents who are strict with routines might raise kids that don't have any routine at all as an act of rebellion.

How our parents diet, exercise, and talk about health in general will also form our own body perceptions. A daughter of a mother who consistently crash diets and works out too hard will likely produce a daughter that does the same. A father that only eats microwave meals or fast food is setting his kids up for doing the same when they become adults. When this happens, it is an insidious issue that we might not even recognize. The things our parents do can seem normal to us, as it is behavior that we learn is standard. By confronting our dieting present, we have to evaluate our past habits.

Be mindful of how you talk about exercise around children. Whether they are your kids or someone else's, never talk about body issues around kids. If you walk around talking about how much you hate your belly flab, you are teaching the kids around you to evaluate their own stomachs, wondering if they, too, have too much belly flab. Kids will be confronted with these body issues in other ways, as it is inevitable. As parents, caretakers, or any sort of role models, we should be teaching our kids how to love their bodies and properly take care of them because they deserve to be healthy, not because they should be skinnier or prettier.

Pregnant Moms Who Exercise Will Likely Give Birth to Healthy Kids

A study was conducted in which one group of pregnant rats were given exercise wheels, while another group of pregnant rats wasn't given anything. Those who used the exercise wheels ended up giving birth to more active babies. The babies of the moms that didn't work out would sit around and not do anything, as opposed to the babies of the moms that were always using an exercise wheel, who would use the wheel themselves. This was true for at least half of the rats born from active mothers. They weren't given anything else, so there weren't any factors to determine the difference in the level of activity other than the environment in which they were raised in the womb.

This exercise was inspired from similar research done on humans, though many scientists wonder if the effects were just because of a mother's influence after birth. Instead of assuming that it was from the active pregnancy, many scientists speculate that the difference in the amount of desire for physical activity is because mothers with active pregnancies are also mothers with active lives. It is clear that their lifestyle and habits can affect children, but the study with the rats proves that it might be on a level different than just the learned behavior.

Even in the womb, our mothers are teaching us how to exercise. We learn before we're even walking how important exercise is in maintaining a high level of physical activity. If a mother is more active while she's pregnant, she's setting her unborn baby up for a future in which it is just generally more active. This means that not only are we affected by the learned habits of our parents, but how we are actually created and grown also determines how much physical activity we let into our life.

Look back on your mother, father, or any other person that helped raise you, biologically or not. Were they active? Did they let that level of activity negatively affect your life? Did they reject exercise and healthy eating at all costs? Did you learn your unhealthy eating habits, or are they just a product of not being taught anything at all? We are taught how to eat and exercise, which means we are also taught *how not* to eat healthy or exercise. We can't fully blame our parents for the way we live now, but it is still important to recognize as it'll help bring us closer to closure with the unhealthy person in our head.

This is good motivation for any woman hoping to get pregnant in the future. Starting a family is a goal for many different people. An important aspect in starting that family is making sure to have a high level of physical activity. Kids require a lot of chasing and lifting. It is much harder for those that are not in shape to look after and give proper attention to active kids. It is also important to be healthy when pregnant with them in order to get them started right away with a healthy lifestyle. After kids are born, parents are also responsible for making sure their kids understand how to live a healthy lifestyle that does not include any bad habits.

Mindfulness Training Helps

Extensive research is being done on the positive effects of mindfulness and meditation. When a person is conscious of their surroundings and what their eating habits might be, they are more aware of the factors that make up for the fundamentals of why they are eating. Mindfulness is an attempt at a person putting emphasis on their surroundings and what's physically happening at any given time. Mindfulness is all about not thinking of the future or ruminating about the past. Reminiscing and planning are not harmful, but doing too much of either thing can certainly be.

Maintaining a diet can be the biggest problem for those who embark on a weight-loss journey. When a person is mindful, they will better be able to control their current situation instead of worrying so much about the past or future. When a person is mindful, they can better control their own thoughts and emotions rather than feeling overwhelmed by all their thoughts. If someone is always anxious about the future, they are going to be very worried about keeping up with their diet. They are taking on feelings of future failure instead of focusing on how to actually prevent that failure in the present moment. When we're not mindful, it can lead to moments of stress and anxiety that will lead to overeating or punishment purging.

The biggest way to be mindful about eating is to not do it while you are doing something else. Instead of sitting down in front of the TV, try to eat at a table where you can talk to someone else. If you focus on the show rather than how much you are eating, you are likely to continually stuff yourself until you are in pain rather than carefully tracking how much you are eating. You might grab a bag of chips when a movie starts, and before you know it, you are only halfway through the movie but all the way through the bag. The best way to be mindful when you eat is to just focus on only eating. This can be more enjoyable when meals are shared as well.

Appreciate the food that you are eating. In order to practice mindful eating, take in every bite slowly and focus on how it makes you feel overall rather than on what you might be doing later. Taste the food and savor each bite. Think of the work that went into creating that meal and the positive effects the food is going to have on your body. When we put an emphasis on this rather than on other things, we eat much slower which means we end up digesting better.

Sometimes, we eat so fast that we still feel hungry, so we end up going back for more. Instead, eat slowly so that you can feel yourself getting full rather than just trying to eat as much as possible. Take a break in between portions in order to ensure you are not just eating because you can. If you eat a lot of food in a quick amount of time, you are just setting yourself up for a night of misery.

Not only does this help someone in their weight-loss journey, but it can have very positive effects on other areas of one's life as well. Being mindful is not important just to shed pounds. It is also crucial to making sure you are actually living in the moment and enjoying your surroundings. Sometimes, eating might be a way to distract ourselves from different forms of pain. If we're mindful of that pain and how to overcome it, we're not only better off in our life in general, but we also eliminate the urge to eat when we aren't hungry.

Portion Control

Some restaurants use large portion sizes to give the illusion that they are giving you more for their money. Fast food restaurants, as well as sit-down chains, will advertise huge portions, boasting about burgers that are a quarter of a pound. This kind of "more for your money" mentality is present in all forms of capitalism, but it is dangerous when it is in terms of food. The larger the drink you get at the movies, the more money you save. Why get a medium when a large is only a quarter more? We think we're getting such a great deal for our money, but really, we just paid a small fee to get twice as many calories as we need.

Studies have proven that individuals given larger portion sizes will eat more even if they don't particularly like the taste of the food. For example, someone might go to the movies and order a small popcorn. The cashier tells them they should get a large, as it is twice as much, but they only have to pay a dollar more. Not thinking, that customer ends up ordering the largest option of popcorn. Then, during the movie, they realize the popcorn is stale and needs salt. Even though they don't like the way it tastes, that customer still eats the entire large bucket because they don't want to waste their money. This kind of mentality manifests itself in other ways and can be incredibly dangerous for anyone that is trying to diet. We have to be aware of how portion promises and promotions trick us into spending more money.

We also feel a need to finish our plates in order to ensure we're getting our money's worth. We go out to eat and order a plate of pasta, and we decide to get the dinner version. It is way too much, but we still eat the last few bites because it is not enough to justify getting a to-go box, but it is also too much to just dump in the trash. We fear wasting our food (that is going to be wasted anyways), so we eat massive portions just to feel better about saving a few dollars.

When you go out to a restaurant, before you even start eating, split it in half. If you get a burger and some fries, cut it in half and separate the fries. Try to eat only half; that way you can take the other half home. If you halve the portion before you even start eating, you allow yourself to see how much you have left, so you enjoy the bites you take, while still making sure you don't eat too much. Then you will still have more for your money by having an entire second meal at home. By getting into this mental habit, we are better able to track our portions both when going out to eat and when serving ourselves at home.

Even take-home packages are way too large. Always check the portions before eating anything. Just because it is handheld and came from a vending machine does not mean you should be eating it all in one sitting. If you look at the nutrition facts, you might realize that drink you have every morning is actually supposed to be three different servings. We allow our portion perspective to become warped because we use packaged food as a standard.

Some people find success in weight loss by just cutting down portions. That is why certain programs, like Weight Watchers, work so well for many different people. Some people might only eat healthy food, yet they can't figure out what it takes to actually lose weight. Eating only vegetables is still unhealthy if you eat pounds of veggies a day. Your body still takes in everything that you eat, storing, using, and wasting every part of that food. Just because it is healthy does not mean it might not still have some fat that your body chooses to store.

Our brains don't see portions, just plates. If only we had the natural biological urge to perfectly portion out meals like we know that we want to eat, many of us would be a lot better off. Unfortunately, some of our eyes are way bigger than our stomachs, and we don't always know what's best for us in terms of portion control. Many animals have to be monitored about how much food they are given, or else they will eat everything in their bowl until it is empty. This is from a natural instinct to load up on food. Some animals in the wild go days without finding another kill, so they make sure to stuff their bodies so they don't go hungry in between meals. We need to be mindful that part of our brains have this kind of instinct as well. It is not as intense as it is for some animals, but we do still have to be incredibly cautious of the urge to clean our plate.

Eating slow is the best way to make sure that you are not overeating. Let your stomach catch up to your mind. Also, always go with tiny portions. This way, if you want seconds, you can go for it! If you cooked a huge serving of pasta, don't load up your plate. It is not as if the pasta is going to disappear while it is sitting in a bowl on your stove. You can always go back and get more! You are also giving yourself the illusion that you are eating more. For example, maybe an average pasta dinner for you is three cups of cooked pasta. Next time you go to eat dinner, start out with just a cup of pasta. Eat slowly, and if you are still hungry, go back for a second round. After that, you will likely not be hungry because the first portion caught up with you. You will also have the idea in your head that you already went for seconds, so you will avoid going up for a third time as it just becomes excessive. You will likely feel full after two cups, even though you have become accustomed to eating three.

Use smaller containers and plates as well. Instead of finding the biggest bowl in your cabinet for your cereal, just use a small cup. If you want a second serving of cereal, you can do so without finishing an entire box in one sitting!

When eating snacks, don't bring the entire container to the couch. Instead, pour your chips into a bowl or cup. If the bag of chips is just sitting next to you on the couch, you are going to eat the whole thing. Instead, if you just fill a cup, when you are done, you will likely just let yourself feel satisfied as you will have to get back up for a second portion.

Chapter 3 – Strategies and Mind Exercises

When we think of weight management, our minds often go to diet and exercise. What's more important than hitting the gym is exercising our brain. If we make sure that the most important organ in our body is taken care of, we can be certain that other healthy habits will soon follow. You can diet, exercise, and do everything else you need to lose weight, but if you continually distract, deflect, or flat out avoid your problems and root issues, you will never find true happiness. The happier you are and the more aware you can be of your mental health, the better it will be in the end which will also lead to an overall better quality of life.

Keep a Journal

Keeping a journey is a healthy habit for many people no matter what their goals, but it's important for someone that wants to lose weight as well. By writing down your different portion measurements and exercise habits, you can better ensure that you'll have a basis for evaluation. When this is done, you can predict future problems that might keep you from your goals by looking back on the days of recorded mistakes or slipups. You can see what kinds of schedules and structures aren't working so you can create better habits in the end. The more extensive your journaling, the better you'll be able to create your own research study of your weight-loss journey, meaning you can share your progress or use it as a structure for future diets.

Avoid the Scale

The biggest issue with weight-loss strugglers comes when they see the number on the scale. Someone that wants to lose ten pounds might get discouraged if they find they only lost nine. Sometimes, people might even have to gain weight before they end up losing a pound. By avoiding the scale altogether, certain failures and disappointments can be avoided as well.

Find a different way to track your progress. You can have monthly weigh-ins, but it shouldn't be something that should be checked once a day. Our weight fluctuates so much throughout our journey that it isn't worth stressing over on a daily basis. Any checking that happens more than once a day is also likely a bad habit; you're using it to distract yourself from a bigger issue.

The Calorie Myth

When many people diet, they focus too much on calories. They'll see that a certain snack pack only has a hundred calories, which means that it's good for you, right? Wrong. When we focus too much on how many calories are in something, we're failing to look at all the other factors that make up that product. Something with zero calories might include harmful chemicals or hidden substances that are bad for us. Something with a ton of calories might be avoided even though it has a large number of vitamins and necessary fiber.

Calories should still be considered, as the more calories you take in, the more you have to burn through exercise. They still shouldn't be a basis for what foods you decide to eat. If you focus too much on calories, you'll end up losing sight of other important issues. Remember that weight loss isn't about numbers. What's on the scale or on the nutrition package is important in making certain measurements, but they shouldn't be the definitive goals that you're creating on your weight-loss journey.

Talk About It

Keeping things in is never good. In fact, it can feel pretty awful. Those that are overweight might find themselves feeling embarrassed about their weight. Maybe they end up making excuses for themselves when they eat certain foods, verbalizing these reasons to others around them as a form of validation. "Oh, I'll just start my diet tomorrow," you might hear someone say as they sneak a few extra cupcakes from the dessert table. This kind of discussion can be counterintuitive. Instead, try talking about the issues and struggles you have rather than about the way you're going to make up for your problems later. You might find that you end up getting some great advice from a person that's going through a similar struggle.

It's important to be a good listener as well. Sometimes, people aren't looking for answers or advice when they're complaining about their issues. It's nice to just have someone to vent to every once in a while. By creating a discussion, you can more easily tackle the issues that are causing problems in your weight-loss journey.

Avoid telling people about your goal before you get on track, however. Talking about your feelings, emotions, and struggles is always a good thing. Sometimes it just takes saying a thing out loud for it to feel real. However, many people set themselves up for failure by sharing their goals too early. Those that post on social media about how they're going to lose weight are actually less likely to follow through with their goals. Stay silent with the majority in the beginning of your journey, confiding in just those you know you can rely on and trust.

Affirmations

Practicing affirmations is an important mindset strategy in weight loss. An affirmation is a type of positive reinforcement that helps in combating negative thoughts. Instead of telling yourself you're "no good" because you didn't follow through with a small goal, you should give yourself an affirmation such as "I am capable of continuing" to remind yourself of how powerful you really are. Below is a list of positive affirmations you should use in order to combat negative thoughts and improve overall encouragement:

1) I can do this. I am capable of losing weight and I have the ability to reach my goals.

2) I am exercising every day and eating healthy as often as possible. I am actually doing what I should be doing in order to achieve my goals.

3) If I can start my journey, I can finish it.

4) I do not need processed foods to feel happy. I can feel the same joy from cooking a healthy meal.

5) I have exercised before and can do it again. It is hard to start, but I know that once I do, I have what it takes to finish my exercise routine.

6) I am healing myself. I have been through challenging times and deserve to feel happy.

7) I am loved and am full of love.

8) I am losing weight to be healthy.

9) I am beautiful no matter what size. Skipping one day at the gym does not mean that I am not beautiful.

10) I am eating healthy food full of nourishment. I can feel the positive change in my body and I know that I only have more to look forward to.

Chapter 4 – Time Management

The most important part of a weight-loss journey is time management. This doesn't mean setting a quick goal and achieving it as fast as possible. It's all about using time properly and understanding how long it takes to actually do something. We set ridiculous goals for ourselves in the hopes that we'll achieve something great, but what ends up happening is, as the end-date approaches, we become overwhelmed and are set up for disappointment. We have to be realistic with our time goals and consider all factors when making different plans.

Practice Patience

Patience is hard to achieve. Anyone that wants to lose weight hopes that they can just jump on the scale after eating a salad and see the number drop by double digits. We have to accept before starting a weight-loss journey that this will never happen. We won't be able to just lose the weight overnight.

Sometimes, patience is hard to have when exercising. Many people find themselves getting bored on treadmills or other machines that require repetitive activity for minutes at a time. Use different exercise methods that you find fun or entertaining, such as a dance class or going on an interesting trail run. If the gym is your only option, use the boring moments on machines as a way to meditate. Clear your head, not thinking of how much weight you want to lose or what else you have to do to get there. Just practice counting or focusing on a quiet place you find peace in, such as a beach or a park. Visualize this in order to find a place of meditation. It'll take practice, but you'll soon find that you can zone out and work hard if you just focus.

There is No Rush

Weight loss takes time; we can't emphasize that enough. Some diets and exercises will help you lose weight quicker than others, but overall, you're going to have to put in a lot of time to lose weight. Remember not to feel too rushed throughout this journey. You have to be strict and consistent to actually see results, but there's no point in forcing yourself into ridiculous time constraints. If you cause yourself anxiety over certain dates, you might feel the need to stress-eat or go through dangerous dieting practices to get there.

Set Small Goals

Instead of looking at a wedding coming up in a couple of months as your goal for losing weight, instead, use that as a small milestone. Many of us get worried looking at the future, thinking of things coming up as the time limits for which we have to lose weight. Maybe it's March and you only have a couple months until swimsuit season. Instead of going on a diet to lose thirty pounds in three months, use the beginning of summer as a small milestone in your journey. Aim, instead, to be healthier and more confident by the time summer comes, rather than giving yourself a ridiculous goal that you don't even know if you can achieve.

Don't Wait for Monday

Many people have an unhealthy perceptive of dieting when looking at certain periods of time. Maybe it's a Tuesday, and so they tell themselves that next Monday is going to be the date to start dieting. In preparation for that date, that same person might make sure to eat all the junk in their house to make sure temptation is removed. But then, by the time Monday comes, something else happens that delays it further.

Even worse, maybe it's Sunday night and you decide that since tomorrow is Monday, you're going to start your diet right now. But then, Tuesday comes, and the diet doesn't start, so you feel discouraged and you count that as just another time that you failed! Don't do this! Instead, set a starting point much further into the future. Find a date two weeks away, whether it's on a Monday, the first of the month, or just a random Wednesday. That way, you can prepare for the official diet-start date. This way, you can practice as the actual date approaches.

For example, your New Year's resolution might be to lose weight. If that's the case, throughout December, you should practice incorporating workout routines a few times a week and experiment with healthy dinners. Then, when January comes around, you have more experience in dieting and are better prepared to actually start your journey than if you had only given yourself a few days to prep.

Something to Tend

Your weight is something to tend. Think of it like a plant. You don't just plant a flower and walk away. The flower will grow, but if you don't go back and make sure to water it, the flower will die. Your journey is a flower. By purchasing this book, you've purchased the seeds. As you read these words, you're reading how to plant the seed and how to make sure that it stays alive. After you've finished the book, it's time to plant the seed. This is done by creating a workout plan and diet.

Once the flower blossoms, you'll have reached your weight-loss goal. Just like the flower, if you abandon your goals and don't tend to your weight-loss journey, you will fall off track and go back into your old lifestyle.

Lifestyle Change

Losing weight isn't just a reduction in numbers. It's a change in the entire way you live your life. There are some people that seem very thin and yet they might be able to eat whatever they want. These people give the illusion that if an overweight person becomes thin, they can then start to eat what they want. That's not how it works, however. Those thin people are just among the handful of individuals that were just born lucky! If you're overweight now, there's a good chance that it's part of your makeup, and weight fluctuations might just be something you have to learn how to manage.

This means you can't just cut out soda for a year, lose fifty pounds, and then start drinking soda again. The weight will come back if you don't manage your habits. That idea can be scary for some people. They might assume that they have to give up soda forever. That doesn't have to be the case. What has to change is just how much soda you can consume. If you drink a Coke a day, you might want to just give the Coke up, hoping you can go back to that behavior after you lose a certain amount of weight.

You have to accept that you can no longer drink a Coke every day if you want to keep up with your weight. Instead, maybe just have soda on weekends, or only when you're going out to eat. Find a way to incorporate the things you desperately love from your past life into your new healthy lifestyle.

Keeping the Weight Off

The part where many people really fall through with their goals is after they actually achieve them! Many people get to their desired weight, see that number, and think they no longer have to keep up with their diet plan. Then, the weight comes back, and the cycle of disappointment has to be lived all over again. Remember that once you reach your first goal, you should set another one. The second might not be as extreme. For example, maybe your first goal is to get down to 180 pounds. Once you do that, you have to come up with something new. That might be getting down to 170 pounds, or it could be something different, such as improving the muscle mass in a certain part of your body. Never stop setting goals. The level of difficulty can fluctuate. But to stay on track and keep the weight off, you have to continually encourage yourself to do better.

Change Things Up

Some people might find that after a year or two of dieting and exercising, they stop losing weight. This can be because their bodies are now used to the healthy behavior. You probably won't ever lose as much weight in a diet as you do at the beginning. Those transformations can be invigorating, but remember that as you continue, it will become a little less drastic.

If you feel you've plateaued in your diet, you should consider changing things up. This might involve trying an entirely new diet, or it could be working out in a different way. Incorporating variety helps to ensure that you'll stick to your goals while also having fun!

Don't Revel in Regret

Once you reach your weight-loss goals, you might find yourself feeling regretful. Maybe you feel remorse over not doing it sooner. You might think to yourself about how if you had started exercising as a teen, it wouldn't be so hard to keep up with the weight now. Don't blame your past self for what they didn't do. Instead, thank them for what they taught you. There is no going back in time. What happened, the decisions we made, and the weight we gained already occurred, and there's no reversing. Instead, we have to look at our past mistakes and use them as lessons.

Remember that you wouldn't be the person you are right now if you hadn't experienced every single thing you did. The more you learn to love yourself, the better you'll be able to forgive the past "you" for all the things they did you wish they hadn't.

It Gets Easier

Always remember that it will get easier. You just have to get into a healthy lifestyle with good habits. The more practice you put into working out, and the more dedicated you are to your diet, the better you'll be able to manage your weight. The first day at the gym is going to be tough. You might be excited to start, but there also might be feelings of fear of judgment and anxiety that you might fail. Don't let anything discourage you from going back. Each and every time you walk through the doors of your gym or decide *not* to eat the candy in the workroom, remember that next time, it's going to get even easier.

The struggle doesn't end. Your legs will always be sore after an intense workout. You'll still sweat through your T-shirts, and you'll still crave all the sweets that caused the weight gain in the first place. Those difficulties don't just disappear. However, the more dedicated you are and the better focus you have on achieving your goals, the easier it gets each and every time.

Conclusion

While many people think that weight loss is about just working out, the most important key to shed the pounds is in your own brain. Our brains are made up of our experiences, the things we were taught, the things we've seen, and the biology of our brains provided by ancestors and our parents. Our brains are the most important organ in our body. Without then, we are just bodies. Our bodies are also important, but if we don't take care of our brain, we can't truly take care of the rest.

Weight-Loss Mindset Review

There are many different steps to losing weight, but finding the right weight-loss mindset requires a few key steps that are important for everyone, no matter if they're on a ketogenic diet or trying out Weight Watchers. In order to achieve a weight-loss mindset, you must:

1) Look inward. What is it about food that makes it so hard to give up?

2) Figure out the role that food plays in your life. Is it a comfort tool for a past trauma?

3) Evaluate the way you were raised. What triggers have been created that might have led to your current behavior? Look at your parents or the people that raised you. How did their dieting behavior affect you?

4) Be easy on yourself. You're not going to reach your goals by belittling yourself along the way.

5) Practice patience. Accept and understand that it's going to be a struggle. Be kind to yourself if something takes longer than you want it to and be forgiving if you have a slipup. It will take time to reach your goals.

Be Proud of Yourself

No matter where you are in your weight-loss journey, at any given time, you should be proud. Over sixty percent of the U.S. population is overweight, so it's not like you're the only one that struggles to diet and exercise. The fact that you even want to change is something you should be proud of. It's not easy, and if it were, everyone would be thin and healthy. Even though you might want to blame yourself for being here in the first place, remember that positive reinforcement is the way you're going to be able to keep up with your goals.

Remember, it is Up to You

You can use different tools, gym memberships, or workout gear to help encourage you to live a healthier lifestyle. At the end of the day, the only thing you can depend on is yourself. Your motivation, desire, and dedication are the only things that's will help you find the life that you've always wanted, and certainly deserve.

WEIGHT LOSS PSYCHOLOGY FOR WOMEN

Powerful Strategies and Motivational Quotes to Ignite your Weight Loss Success!

FELICIA URBAN RN, MSN

Introduction

At any given moment, you can walk into a store and find a section dedicated to weight loss. If you go to your local grocery store, they will have an aisle full of protein shakes and meals, weight loss supplements, and meal replacements. You can go to the soda section and see diet soda, the chip aisle and see baked chips, and the frozen area to find rows and rows of diet meals. If you go to a bookstore, you'll see an entire section dedicated to weight loss books. When going to a clothing store, there will be sections dedicated to workout gear.

The weight loss industry is approaching a $70 billion market. It is safe to say that if weight loss wasn't an issue in our society, the economy would look a lot different. All of the things mentioned in the first chapter are ways that various people are profiting off our (the average person's) struggle. We are sold addictive fast food just to take addicting weight loss supplements so that we can go online and become addicted to our social media pages, which are filled with airbrushed models. So many companies are so dependent on our desire to lose weight that if no one cared what they looked like or how healthy they were, these companies would go out of business. It is important that we recognize the power this weight loss industry has over the many individuals struggling with their body weight.

Even if everyone was at their ideal weight and had perfect health, these industries would still be trying to sell you their products, making us consistently feel as though our bodies aren't good enough. Every weight loss product you see will state how they are "the one," or that their brand holds the secret of weight loss that everyone has been waiting for. Pills promise that if you take them, you'll lose inches off your waist. There are shakes that say that if you drink that instead of an actual meal, you'll have the body of your favorite model. We have to understand that the secret to our weight loss is never going to lie within a pill, supplement, or meal replacement. The key to getting the weight off, and keeping it off, exists within our own minds. Sure, some things can help in your weight loss, but you can't just expect to think with the same mind that caused the weight gain, take a pill, and instantly lose weight. Unfortunately, it is just not that easy. Once you get through the hard part, overcoming your original mindset, you will see that you can't really go back. When you get into the right weight loss mindset and alter your perspectives and motivations, then you likely won't go back to the way things used to be as easy as it was to do with other diet plans.

This book is a great stand-alone book, but it also enhances and works exceptionally well with the first book Weight Loss Psychology For women: Kick the fat Girl Out of your Head and Lose the Weight

Permanently! In the last book, we went over the right mentality that you need to get in and all the factors you've experienced in your life that might have caused you to get into an unhealthy mindset in the first place.

Throughout this book, we're going to talk about your mindset now, and the powerful strategies that helped me to keep up with the motivational headspace that I created while coming up with the first book.

A lot of the reason that you might struggle with weight loss is because of the physiological things that you've experienced in the past. The first book goes more over your upbringing and how that affected your mentality, and in this book, we're going to be focusing on the "now." While reflecting on our past is crucial if we want to look deep into ourselves, we can't get stuck thinking about how life used to be. We need to put an emphasis on what's going on right now so that we can make sure we are moving forward and not letting the things that are only memories now consume what time we have.

We will still get into those topics here for readers that haven't checked out the last book, but for a more in-depth look at our past trauma look at the first book. We will go over some triggers, and the most important factors of the last book, but it will be in a refreshing review for those that have already read, and quick enlightenment for the individuals that are coming here first.

I encourage you to also purchase the audio version as the brain learns positive habits the best by incorporating many modes of learning; hearing, reading, etc. This would be great to listen to when working out, having a tough day, needing encouragement, and also as a positive way to start the day. We are going to provide you with the information that you need to make your head prepared for the journey that is to come. I'm also going to share many quotes with you that I have found to be helpful in my journey. Some of these quotes are from others that have lost weight themselves. Many of the quotes are just from other basic resources as well, that relate not just to this weight loss journey but also to everything in life. you will find that not only will it be easier for you to lose the weight and keep it off, but also the other challenges you have in your life through relationships and work will improve too.

I want to remind you now and throughout the book that most diets work if followed but that mindset is the critical component. This won't be the last book in the series either, as the next one will go over the keto diet and how that can really help drive your weight loss success. You might have tried diet after diet, pill after pill, meal after meal, and nothing works. That is because it is not your body, but your mind. You were capable of putting on the weight, so you are going to be capable of losing it. You don't' have to search the pill or meal replacement aisle to find the one that works for you. Instead, you have to find the right mindset. We will take you through all the steps necessary to solidify what we learned in the last book, and promote the mindset needed now.

Chapter 1 – Enhance Your Motivation

"Of course, motivation is not permanent. But then, neither is bathing; but it is something you should do on a regular basis." — Zig Ziglar1

Your journey is going to start with your motivation level. Many things are possible, but it feels like almost nothing is when you are lacking motivation. Getting out of bed morning after morning, trying to find the strength to make it through the day can feel as hard as trying to climb a mountain on some days. Motivation can be found in many different things, but it will always come from our minds. What we're passionate about, the things that really matter, those are what motivates us to make it through the day.

The first thing you are going to want to do to motivate you is to change your attitude into a positive one. When we look at the world through a gray lens, we can easily see everything as terrible. When you hate one thing, that hate starts to grow and can spread into other parts of your life. We can't look at life through rose-colored glasses either, because we don't want to make ourselves ignorant to reality. We have to look at the world, at our life, head on, as it is in an objective way. When we can do this, it will be much easier to take on the new things that present themselves to you each and every day.

Give yourself time to prepare to be motivated too, not just time to start the weight loss. First, you have to get in the right mindset. Then, you can prepare for your meal plan and exercise regimen before starting. If you try to force yourself into it, you might sometimes make it even harder to get started.

As humans, we like to be independent. Not everyone is interested in being told what to do and we sometimes seek to be defiant in ways, even against ourselves. Sometimes in our heads, the things we're being told to do won't be our own ideas and can instead simply be the pressures of society, our peers, and our parents. Their voices can still get so deep in our heads that we will mistake them for our own and can easily get frustrated with what we're telling ourselves.

It can seem like an internal battle when you are trying to get motivated. There's the part of you that knows what you have to do, and then there's the voice that's telling you to just not do it. To just sit around and wait for tomorrow. Motivation is all about silencing that voice and building one of encouragement.

Don't allow any regret into your life or into the future. Regret can be such a wasted emotion. At the end of the day, it is not. There is a psychological purpose for regret. It causes us to look back on our mistakes and question our motives for doing certain things. Regret can teach us how to be better in the future. However, too much regret can lead to a lot of time wasted. There are some individuals that will be so regretful over certain decisions that it consumes their entire life. If you want to move forward and be motivated, not just about weight loss but with everything in your life, then you have to learn how to let go of regret. Feeling it in the first place isn't wrong, but don't entertain it anymore. Think of it like someone that you pass at the grocery store, someone that that you want to still is respectful towards even though you aren't very fond of him or her. Instead of talking to them and inviting them out to dinner, simply smile at them and keep walking. This is how we have to learn to process all feelings of regret, and emotions of guilt and shame as well. Simply let it passes, but do not allow it to stay past its welcome.

You are the person that you are right now because of the life that you've lived. It can be so easy to think, "Oh I should have done this," or "if only I had gone with the other option." However, if we hadn't made that one choice, then our lives would be incredibly different than what they are now. Each thing we've experienced, the decisions we've made and the thoughts that we've had, these are all like ingredients that go into what makes us who we are. When you can learn to love yourself and the person that you've become, then it will be easier to build that motivation because you'll let that guilt and regret losing.

Look at what motivates you right now, at this very second. What's the first thing that comes to mind? Maybe it is wanting to make a loved one proud or providing for your child. Perhaps your motivation is getting your bills paid or simply making your next meal. Whatever it is, this can tell you a lot about what drives you in this life. When you can become aware of all the motivating factors in your life, it will be a lot easier to use these images and ideas when you are struggling in certain situations. If nothing comes to mind at all, then it is time to do some soul searching. At the very least, wanting to make ourselves happy should be a motivator. Feeling good and looking better is all I need to motivate me on some days; however, others require a little more work.

Honestly, sometimes food was a motivator for me. I would tell myself that if I could avoid fast food all week and eat healthy Monday-Friday, that Saturday, I could go crazy. I told myself it didn't' matter if I wanted to drive myself through Taco Bell, Wendy's, and KFC all in one week. Whatever I decided for Saturday would be fine, as long as I stayed resilient against my cravings for Monday-Friday. If I was struggling on Wednesday and just wanted to skip the salad I brought to work and walk to the fast food joint across the street, I would remind myself that I could get it on Saturday. When I would diet in the past, I would think that I had to cut all bad food out for the time being. It would drive me crazy! Eventually, I realized that I had to give myself looser restrictions and reminding myself that it wouldn't be too long before I could have fast food again helped to keep me motivated throughout the week, rather than constantly thinking about the food that I wanted.

What would end up happening was that I felt so good about myself for eating healthy all week that I wouldn't want to ruin my streak so I would keep up the diet. I would get to Saturday and think to myself that I had done so well all week, why ruin it now? I might still occasionally go out to dinner with my family on the weekends and get something that isn't great for me, but then this was a reward. I realized that motivation would breed more motivation. The easier it was for me to get started with the things I want and stay focused on my goals, the more this strengthened my willpower. There are always going to be hard days, but I just remind myself that this is part of the process.

"No one wakes up in the morning and says, 'I want to gain 150 pounds and I will start right now!" — Tricia Cunningham[2]

Your Dream Outfit

"Weight loss doesn't begin in the gym with a dumbbell; it starts in your head with a decision." — Toni Sorenson[3]

Some people will put pictures of their celebrity icons on their fridge, or maybe even their mirror, so that they see them when they wake up. You need motivation that will help you picture yourself in your future, not someone else's body and journey. If your main motivation is done through comparing yourself to others, then that's not going to be healthy in the long-run. Instead, it might drive you to eat more because you are feeling bad about yourself, in more of a fragile state where you are going to decrease motivation levels. The thing about celebrity bodies is that if they aren't photo shopped, then they were still achieved through trick lighting and a team of makeup artists, as well as a personal trainer and shopper that gives them all the tools needed to lose weight. Most of us women are doing this on our own, so we have to stay realistic.

If you are 5 feet tall and you put a Victoria's Secret model on your fridge, that's not going to do you any good. We all have different bodies, and even if you were at your healthiest body weight, you might still not look anything near to the person that you are comparing your body to. Some of us are naturally curvier as well, while others might be stick-thin. You might have larger breasts and hips, or a bigger shoulder structure than many thinner models on the runway. We can't expect our bodies to look like theirs if the structure and height aren't the same, so using other people's pictures is never a good idea. It can just make you feel worse about yourself because you might get below your healthy weight and still not look like the other person, so you will still be disliking your body.

Right now, think of what your ultimate dream outfit would be. Whether it is a slim-fitting dress, or a cute crop-top and some butt-lifting high waist jeans, think of an outfit that you want to be able to look totally cute in. This is going to be your biggest motivator when you are getting started. You will be able to actually see yourself in this dress and be able to look at it with your own body, not just what someone else might look like. Be realistic with your sizing as well. Only go down a few sizes, somewhere that you would still feel good about yourself getting into. If you are a size 24 right now and you buy a size 0 dress, that's unrealistic. That could take years to get into, and there's a good chance that your body structure still wouldn't be able to slip into a 0. This is a small size and people that are a size 0 and have a healthy body weight are usually shorter, so be realistic. A size 16 dress would probably be a good place to start if you are currently at a 24. And if you are a size 16 now, then a size 10 would be good. Make sure you are aiming for something in between what your size is now, and what half of that size would be, give or take a number.

Try to not pick a bikini or something that would make you feel uncomfortable. A bikini or swimsuit can be good for some people, but swimwear can be triggering for many women, especially those that have continuously struggled with their weight. Pick something that you would wear now at your comfort level. If you try to push yourself too hard, you could end up making yourself afraid of what might happen and could even self-sabotage.

Hang this outfit somewhere that you will see it every single day. I put it on the back of my bedroom door so that I could see it every day when I woke up and every night before I fell asleep. It would help me to remind myself of all that I wanted to achieve and give me the strength and encouragement in the morning to not give up on the thing that I wanted the most. Make sure that you are giving yourself the proper time to reach this goal as well. If you try to fit into something 10 sizes smaller after 2 months, you are just going to end up disappointing yourself.

Studies on Habit

We all have different habits that we do. Some people have a habit of working out every day, others have a habit of eating a candy bar every night. Whatever it is, there are certain things that we do ritualistically. Sometimes, we don't even realize that what we are doing is a habit. Our brains can become so accustomed to doing the same thing over and over again that we won't always recognize when we've adopted behavior that is consistent and harder to break. Instead, we have to look at others to remind us of our habits and point out the things that we consistently do.

Habit forming actually starts within the neurology of our brains. When you are learning something, you take it in and process it in a certain way. Your brain takes the information and decides if it wants to store it in the long-term or short-term memory. You learn what you can from each experience and then your brain moves onto other things. It does this when learning or doing all new things. After repeatedly taking in that same information, your brain will no longer process it the same. Your brain just won't give it the same amount of energy. It becomes second nature because your brain doesn't think there's anything valuable to get from it. For example, you might have a habit of going for a walk every day. On that first walk, your brain took in that information, and you noticed everything new. The houses along the path, the marks in the sidewalk, the biggest trees, you noticed all this kind of stuff. Then, as you kept going on the same walk, on that same route, your brain stopped looking for something new. It became a habit.

Habits will give us the ability to put our attention on something else[4]. If we were constantly alert and paying attention to all the details of everything we see and experience, then it can be very overwhelming for our brains. We can even go through sensory overload. We need to take a break sometimes and just do the mindless things, so our consciousness isn't always working so hard. However, if everything becomes a habit, then our brains will also stop evolving and growing.

We have to start recognizing our habits if we ever want them to change. This can be hard, but it just requires you to be mindful throughout the day. before doing anything, ask yourself why you're doing it. Even if it's simply going to the bathroom. As you stand up from the couch to go pee once you get that feeling in your bladder, recognize what you are doing, why you're doing it, and the motivation behind it. When we can practice mindful living in all aspects of our lives, then it becomes easier to do so more naturally. Motivation can build the desire to change your intentions, but it is only up to you to actually change the outcome. You might get the fantasy or exciting idea to lose the weight and go on a diet. However, actually going through with that will require you to recognize and break your worst habits.

Just like you took a little while to form a habit, it is going to take a bit to get it to go away. You won't be able to just stop the habit overnight. Your brain was trained to do this! Have you ever tried to brush your teeth with the opposite hand? It can be challenging! Remember that you aren't just habitual for no reason. You can look deep inside yourself to see what drives you and do your best to break those bad habits.

Research on Motivation

We need motivation to do literally anything. A lot of times, we don't realize the motivation behind certain actions. How many times have you reflected on something you've done and thought, "Why on Earth did I just do that?" Though we feel like we're in charge often, there are a lot of times when it feels like we have almost no control at all. This is because sometimes, our subconscious will think it knows what's best for us better than we would of ourselves. The better we can understand our own motivation on an individual level, the easier it will be to create those feelings of encouragement within ourselves. Those that struggle with weight loss aren't the only ones who are concerned with motivation either. Since it is so relevant in all aspects of life, we have scientific research that allows us insight into what might drive our most basic desires.

We have two different kinds of goals when it comes to motivation, mastery and performance[5]. On one hand, you might desire to achieve something because you want to master that task. You want to be the best person to complete the goal. On the other hand, you might want to outperform someone else. Either way, your motivation will come from one of these two categories.

Our motivations are usually sparked by the desire for reward, competition, and curiosity. When there is something waiting for you at the finish line, then it can motivate you to do better.

If you want to compete with others or prove someone wrong, that can be a key component to motivation as well. When we are simply curious about something and want to know more, that will motivate our curiosity and cause us to look deep within ourselves to fulfill our greatest goals.

Basically, we don't know exactly what can define motivation or cause it in some individuals. At the end of the day, it's going to be up to you to define what it is that drives your motivation. It seems that motivation that is planted there by others doesn't work as effectively as the motivation that works within us.

Someone might call you "fat," so you feel bad and think about how you want to diet. However, that won't always be enough to take you all the way. The best way to motivate yourself is to look inward and see what you want to do to make you happy and help you achieve your personal dreams.

Your Reason for Motivation

Finding a solid reason to lose weight is something that's going to be very important in your journey. On one hand, you won't want to do it just for other people. This is something that you have to do for yourself. If you want to make your spouse, children, peers, parents, or anyone else proud, that's great! But you have to remember that what will matter most in this journey is making yourself proud.

Competition can be helpful, but at first, you just need to focus on yourself, especially if this has been a long journey for you. If you're too competitive, then you might make yourself feel bad. Competition should be fun and encouraging, like doing a small race with a friend. If you base your life around it and only find worth in beating other people, then that's going to be harmful to your perspective on yourself, making it even more challenging to lose the weight and keep it off.

Don't make your motivation be to look "hot" or to be skinny and thin. This is a lot of people's goals. They will measure their success by how skinny they might be looking. This isn't enough to keep you going, however. If this is your only goal, then it could even lead to you taking dangerous measures to try and achieve those goals. Your motivation should be to get healthy. If you switch your perspective from wanting the skinniest body to wanting to be healthy inside and out, then you've already started to love yourself.

We've spent a lot of time in a place where we didn't like our bodies, and that has become a habit. We are used to the skin we are in, whether we like it or not. Just wanting a different body won't always be enough of a motivation. Instead, you should desire to feel as good as possible.

Look at all the ways that being unhealthy has affected your life, not the way that being overweight has. For me, I hated being out of breath when I walked up the stairs. I was tired of never finding anything that fit my body in stores, always having to shop from a limited plus size section. I hated that I couldn't play tag with my kids, and there were sometimes that my clothes even ripped because of my size. I would see a fragile looking chair, or something with minimal support, and become fearful that my body alone would crush it.

I felt like a burden like my body was too big and that I took up too much space. For so long, I wanted to be skinny just so I looked good, never caring about how I felt physically and mentally. I realized that I needed to simply focus on making myself feel better rather than look better. Luckily, the second part came along on its own, but only after I learned to love myself and get into the right mindset.

1) Ziglar, Z. (2010). <u>Raising Positive Kids in a Negative World.</u>
2) Cunningham, T. & Skolnik, H. (2010). <u>The Reverse Diet.</u>
3) Sorenson, T. (2019). <u>The Great Brain Cleanse.</u>
4) Society for Personality and Social Psychology. (2014). <u>How we Form Habits, Change Existing Ones.</u>
5) Murayama, K. (2019). <u>The Science of Motivation.</u>

Chapter 2 – Never Give Up!

"Everything can be taken from a man but one thing: the last of the human freedoms—to choose one's attitude in any given set of circumstances, to choose one's own way." — Viktor E. Frankl[1]

If you are reading this, we can almost guarantee that you have tried to diet before but didn't find any success. There are some things that we are taught to look for on our own. When you feel sick, you can go to the store and get some Tylenol or Nyquil to make you feel better. If you're cold, you grab a blanket from your closet. When you hate your body, what are you supposed to do? We aren't as commonly taught the methods for remedying a distaste with our own bodies, so we will often grasp at whatever we can to try and find a solution for the body that we feel so uncomfortable in.

Before getting started, we have to accept that right now, there's almost a %100 chance that you will have a slip-up, failure, or moment of weakness. If we try to go into this pretending that we are perfect creatures, we will never succeed. If we try to go into this thinking that we are capable of perfection at all, we will never succeed. This is because there is no standard of perfection. A person that seems as though they have reached all of their skills will always seek something greater. We are inherently looking for more. It's consumption that will never stop, so we need to understand that we will never fully achieve a level where we are complètely satisfied with every aspect of our life. That being said, it's also important to address the fact that we need to learn to be comfortable with imperfection. When it comes to weight loss mindset, this is especially true for accepting moments of weakness when we might give into temptation.

Don't look at these moments as times that you give up. I've had so many days where I said, "Today is the day I diet." I would go into it successful for a certain time period. Sometimes it meant an entire month, other times it would simply be through my breakfast and lunch. No matter what happened, I would always have a moment where I would give in. I would order a pizza, go through the drive-thru, eat a tub of ice cream, or do whatever it was that threw me off track for my diet at that time. Then I would think to myself, "well I already failed, so what's the point of trying anymore?" I gave up. Even if I had gone 30 days eating nothing but my leafy greens, whole wheats, and organic fish, I would eat one candy bar and lose all hope for the future of my diet. This kind of mentality was toxic! Sure, that one candy bar wasn't great for me. But that could have been it. I could have gone 1o more days back on track with my diet, but instead, I threw in the towel because I had one minor mishap. We have to stop this kind of thinking right now. Mess-ups are going to happen, and we need to be prepared for them. We will cover all the methods of preparation in the next chapter, but for now, we are going to go over the importance of allowing yourself the freedom to make mistakes.

Sometimes we start to create so much hope around achieving our goals that we end up living in the fantasy rather than reality. I could sit for hours thinking about the perfect body that I wanted, how good I might look in a certain dress, or all the things I could accomplish if I were "skinny." What would happen is that I would sit there for so long, maybe watching TV, scrolling through social media, or just daydreaming while looking out the window imagining what could be, all the while wasting the time that could be spent on actually achieving that dream.

Don't wait around for something to happen. It's so easy to wait for tomorrow because it's not real. What we think is going to happen tomorrow never will. There's an old quote that states how whenever we make a plan, our god, fate, or whatever else you might believe religiously and spiritually laughs. If everything turned out the way that we expect it to, life would be so boring. Tomorrow will happen, but the idea we have for tomorrow is completely fabricated. We can't wait around. We can't just hope that tomorrow is going to be the day that we're motivated. If you're unhappy now, you can't expect that you're not going to be unhappy tomorrow. If we're miserable with our surroundings, then it's going to keep being that way until we do something about it. Those who live in happiness, who exude gratitude for the "now," are those that have realized that they are the ones in charge of every action that they take. We can't control what others might do, what happens in the world, or every other thing that gets thrown our way. We can, however, decide whether or not we are going to take charge over our lives and quit waiting around for something magical to happen. You are the one holding the mysticism. Success exists within your own hands.

Stay the Course

"Do not stop thinking of life as an adventure. You have no security unless you can live bravely, excitingly, imaginatively; unless you can choose a challenge instead of competence." — Eleanor Roosevelt[2]

Let us tell you right now that getting started is probably going to be the hardest part of it all. Think of it like rowing a boat. Before you even get in the boat, you have to make sure you're wearing the right thing, have the proper supplies, and know how to even get into a boat in the first place. Once all of that has been established, it's time to put the boat in the water and climb in. When I got in my first canoe, I didn't know how important balance was and I completely tipped it over! If this happens, you have to get right back in and start over again. Once you're inside the boat, then it's time to paddle. That can be hard at first, especially if you're not the only one on board. However, after those first few strokes of the canoe, you can start easily gliding down the river, stream, or

73

wherever else it is that you're going. The hardest part was getting started, but once that's happened, it's so much easier to stay afloat. If you've never been on a boat and have no idea what I'm talking about, picture that feeling of cutting something, usually wrapping paper, and your scissors start gliding along making the perfect cut. The hardest part is always going to be getting started in the first place.

It can be scary to have to really put yourself out there and try for a goal that you've always wanted. For me, I struggled with my weight all my life. Actually, achieving a body that I wanted and desired seemed like such a fantasy that I never really realized how great it can feel to accomplish. We build up the idea of succeeding with that goal so much that we can sometimes lose sight of what it means to actually gain it. Imagine all the people out there in the online dating world who never actually meet the other person. They might go years "dating" someone without ever actually meeting them. Though they might talk every day, actually meeting them can be scary because the idea of who they are has become more built up than the person that actually exists. The same kind of thinking goes when it comes to the vacations we go on. The anticipation can sometimes be the exciting part. We have to stop thinking like this when it comes to dieting. Don't live in your fantasy. Actually, reach out and achieve the dream that you've been waiting for.

If we had succeeded the first time we tried, look at how much success we could have achieved. I can't even try and count how long I tried different diets and methods of weight loss before actually realizing the importance of weight loss psychology. I know for sure that it was at least years. It took over a year to lose the weight, so I know that I could have got it off much quicker if I would have just stuck to the methods I tried in the first place. However, this regretful mindset isn't going to be helpful in moving forward. I didn't make it through the first time. I messed up and I did things in a way that I wish would have gone down differently. However, it was those "failures," those moments where I didn't do my best that helped me learn about myself and be the person that I've wanted to become all along.

Sometimes, we might even feel like it is too late. For a while, I thought, "Why even bother? I've tried for so many years and nothing worked, so I may as well just be satisfied with the life I have." I'm going to tell you right now, whether you're 18 or 80, achieving your dreams is never too late. Don't' ever stop trying to get what you want. The moment that we let ourselves live by this mentality; we have stopped living. You might say, 'what's the point," often, but as soon as we really buy into this idea, we have given up on ourselves and our futures. Don't let this happen. There is always something that will change your life in ways you never expected. You might have met a friend in a strange way, or maybe you stumble upon a song you like by changing the radio station to a different channel. No matter how insignificant, life-changing moments can happen within the blink of an eye. Never underestimate your future. It can hold so much more power than you can even fathom at the moment.

Look back on your life from the past six months. Wouldn't it have felt better now if you would have at least done the bare minimum rather than not doing anything at all? There were a lot of times that I had an "all or nothing," mentality. I would think I either had to commit myself %100 to weight loss and healthy food, or I had to eat like a total glutton. What I didn't' realize, however, is that some things can happen slowly. Simply going for a walk every day wasn't going to take me from a size 24 to a size 2, but it would be a whole lot better than sitting on the couch for that 20 minutes. Whatever it might be, the smallest thing you can do to contribute to your health, whether it's mental or physical, is a lot better than not doing anything at all.

Starting Over is Harder Than Picking It Back Up

Since the beginning is the hardest, trying to redo the beginning over and over again is going to be incredibly challenging. Back to my story about letting one candy bar determine my fate, pushing through that moment and continuing with my diet rather than quitting and starting over weeks later is a lot easier. Though it seems like we have to take this moment as a failure and give up all hope, in reality, we can simply take any "slip up" as a learning experience and push forward toward a better future. Imagine the journey it takes to ride in a canoe again. If you tipped the canoe, you wouldn't just take it back to the shore and quit, only to try and do it just a few minutes later again. You simply have to flip the canoe back over and keep moving forward. Progress is progress, no matter how big or small. Next time you feel like giving up, just move forward, because it's a lot easier than trying to start all over again later on.

You will have moments where you do things you wish you didn't, and sometimes you might simply feel like a failure. This is just our inner voice letting our anxiety get the best of us. A lot of times, I would tell myself I was a failure. I would say I wasn't good enough and feel like I couldn't do a single thing that was right. I realized one day that no one has ever actually told me that I was a failure. There have been plenty of people that underestimated me, some that have let me down, and a few that have actually said hurtful things to me. However, the person that has been the cruelest to me is myself. No one ever blatantly called me a failure, but I said that to myself plenty of times. Why is it so easy for me to be so damaging to my self-esteem and not as easy to drive my motivation? There is actually scientific evidence that backs up some of the reasoning behind why we might be so hard on ourselves. As animals, we are always looking for improvement. It is a natural instinct to look for the next meal, a better place to settle down location-wise and to find the optimal mate. We are constantly seeking more because it is what is built into our brain. We don't focus on the good and instead store that as a memory. You remember that tacos taste good, but you're still on the quest for the perfect taco. We can't make ourselves feel bad for wanting more. We do have to be mindful about our satisfaction levels and remember to be mindful with the good things that already surround us, including all the qualities that make us unique, valuable individuals.

Don't ever quit! By quitting, we're only making things harder in the end. Even if what we're going through is challenging, finishing out is always better than simply giving up. When we quit, not only do we destroy everything that we've worked for, but we've also validated our fears. We've proven to ourselves that the doubts we had in the first place were just, so it sets us up to be more skeptical of our capabilities in the first place. If you failed once, then your mind reminds you that you can fail again, so we become less hopeful and more disappointed as time goes on. On top of that, it becomes harder to be motivated. We become sick of getting disappointed. It hurts to be disappointed, so our brains will naturally try to avoid this, keeping us from trying things that actually could improve our lives.

In addition to these feelings, we will also find challenges in quitting because we put less value on our goals. If you simply give up on something, then it starts to make you think that maybe it wasn't so worth it in the end. When we give up and give into temptation, then we create this mentality in our head that failing is better than achieving what we were actually trying to gain in the first place.

Imagine if you would have broken up with your significant other/spouse or ended a friendship after one small fight. We'd likely have far fewer people in our lives. This is because we work through the issues, and most of the time, come out stronger in the end. We have to start looking at our relationship with weight loss like we would any other partnership in our lives. You put in half the effort, and you will get something in return. When things are tough, you just have to try harder. Not every moment will be perfect, but overall, the good will always outweigh the bad.

The idea of failing is scary. You can easily start to think of the worst possible scenario when you fail. It can be easier to live in a life of simple comfort than to try and do something scary that could potentially, maybe, perhaps, involve failing. Don't let this idea scare you! Most of the time, even the worst-case scenario isn't as scary as what we build it up to be in our minds. Though you will face some challenges, remember that it's going to carry you to the places that you need to be in the end.

The Journey is Worth it in the End!

"Incredible change happens in your life when you decide to take control of what you do have

The idea that I will regret not doing something more than I will regret doing it plays in my head over and over again whenever I'm questioning what I want to do next. Even if it is meeting a friend out for drinks when I'm already in my pajamas at home. I think about how I don't want to get up to change, I don't want to have to get out of bed, put on pants, and walk or drive to that place. I don't feel like changing my social mode from interacting with the people on my TV to talking to actual humans in the real world. But then I think about the times that I have gone out. I've had so many conversations with people that changed my perspective, inspired me to do something, or taught me something that I never would have learned on my own. It might have been hard to get there in the first place, but it's so worth it in the end.

Continuing is going to feel much better at the end than quitting will, simple as that. When you quit, you set yourself up with all the ideas of what could have happened. Just like we replay the fantasy of "what could be" in our minds over and over again, we play the thought of "what could have been" just as often. You might go over the worst-case scenario in your head, but you will also think about the best-case scenario just as often. You will play in your mind all the amazing things you would have accomplished if only you would have stuck to your diet. We have to be realistic with this, however. You need to make sure that you are doing the best to stay grounded in reality so that you can find the motivation actually required to make it through your journey.

Think about it like you would if you were trying to practice for the Olympics. You are not just going to be great on the first day of practice. It takes days and days and weeks and weeks and months and months of practice! If it could happen all within a few moments, then everyone would have a gold medal by now. it's going to be an upward battle, but what's waiting at the top is going to be incredible. When you achieve your goals and make it through this crazy journey, not only are you fulfilling the desires that you set to reach in the first place, but you're also opening a new aspect of your life that you never would have imagined. The feeling I got when I hit 90 pounds lost was amazing because I hit my target, I reached my goal. That was great. Knowing that I accomplished *a goal*, not just *my goal*, felt so good that I wanted more. I craved the feeling I would get when I reached that next milestone.

Imagine your most exciting action movie, one you keep going back to. Perhaps it's the exciting adventures of Harry Potter, or maybe you're more of a Star Wars girl. Whatever it is, these characters, Luke and Harry, they go through a journey. They make some mistakes and have moments where things didn't work out perfectly, but they kept going. These are fictional characters so it's not going to be as hard for them obviously, but it's still a story that we can admire. Perseverance and dedication are like the life forces that are going to take you right to the place that you want, that you deserve. It will feel better knowing that you actually accomplished something than it will to have actually lost the weight!

Journaling

Create a journal to show your mental progress. For me, someone who likes to express their creativity, this was the fun part. I picked out a cute journal I liked and invested in some colorful pens and markers. Each and every single day, I would spend some time in my journal making sure that I would write down the daily successes of the day. this would include how much I slept, what I ate, the things I felt, and the lessons that I learned. Some days the entries were longer than others. I would forget one day but then I would just write in it the next. Though I found benefits in journaling for tracking my progress, it was also helpful in keeping mindful. Journaling meant that I would take time out of my day to relax and self-reflect. If you aren't a daily journal type at least do a weekly recap.

Use this to revisit times you overcame temptation and rough patches! When I was having a good day and successfully avoided any temptations, I would look back on it on my most challenging days, during the times that were really testing me, and have the basis for the mentality that I needed to seek the level of motivation required to get me through. When I was feeling really bad about myself, I was able to write these feelings down as well. Then, when I head a more positive, clearer mind, I could really evaluate those rough patches so that I would know what caused them, how to get out of that headspace, and what to do to prevent another negative episode.

This is very helpful to pinpoint and overcome triggers. When you are triggered, you don't always realize it. Sometimes, you might go through a day and feel so stressed out, having no idea what's causing all your flooding feelings of emotion. However, if you journal, then you can take the moment to look back on those triggers and determine exactly where they came from and what it might have been that caused them.

Weight loss can be similar to a chess game with yourself, strategize ahead by learning and preparing for your weaknesses. Your journal can be like your playbook. Sometimes, analyzing things numerically helped as well. I would rate my mood on a 1-10 scale every day. Then, I could see that on one day I was an 8, another a 5, some days a 3, and most of the time, I would fall somewhere around 7. I could see exactly what it was that might have caused me to trickle so close to 0, and better find a way to work through that later on.

Your journal can be whatever you want it to be. You can have long entries, letters to yourself, and lists on what you want for the future, and simple "dear diary," entries. You can also include images, such as sketches for the future, collages that are filled with goal pictures, and vision boards that give you inspiration. Whatever it is that you choose, that is completely fine. Try to avoid sharing your journal as well. In the beginning, I would want to take pictures of my journal or show friends. What I found then, later on, was that I was trying to make my journal look good. I wanted it to be something that would impress others. This ruined the point. It took it away from myself and instead gave the power to people that didn't really care that much anyway. Make a journal for yourself. Sharing your journey can be helpful, and we'll get into that later, but you need to make sure you are keeping personal records that only you have access to.

Triggers

We talked a lot about trauma and triggers in the last book, so we will just do a quicker recap in this section. It's important to recognize anything in this life that might trigger us. When you are triggered, it takes you back to the mindset you experienced when initial trauma was felt. Oftentimes, we think of triggers and PTSD as a soldier coming back from the war. They might hear a loud bang sound and think that a bomb is going off, so they can become defensive and fall into an attack mode, ready to be combative with others. This isn't the case. Sometimes, triggers can be very small. I've known a lot of people who yelling was their trigger, so when someone yelled at them, they would instantly shut down and not react as a defensive mechanism.

Triggers can also be anything that is going to elicit the feeling of wanting to go back to unhealthy behavior. An alcoholic might be triggered by the simple sight of a beer can smashed on the sidewalk as they walk home at night, causing them to stop at a liquor store and binge drink the rest of the night. When you have to confront something challenging, it can trigger your brain to a dark place.

A trigger could be walking by a bakery. My triggers are times of stress, especially if I have to cook but don't feel like it. I will think over and over again about how I don't want to have to preheat the oven and get my baking sheets ready, cook all the different parts, serve it, and wash all the dishes. That can be such a struggle on some days. It triggers me to order a pizza, and then I'm left feeling bad about myself, in a headspace much worse than if I would have just cooked an actual homemade meal in the first place.

Triggers aren't just with weight loss either. They could be something completely unrelated. For example, going on a bad date could be a trigger that makes you want to eat an entire cake. You might not experience a trigger directly related to your weight, but it could be something that elicits a feeling of wanting to participate in a behavior that causes unhealthy habits.

When we can pinpoint our triggers, we can either avoid them or come up with a successful strategy and try to conquer them. If you want to learn more about your childhood trauma and how to identify and overcome your triggers then we highly suggest that you check out the first book in this series!

1) Frankl, V. (1946). <u>Man's search for meaning.</u>
2) Roosevelt, E. (2018). <u>Autobiography of Eleanor Roosevelt.</u>
3) Maraboli, S. (2014). <u>Life, the truth, & being free.</u>

Chapter 3 – Being on Top of Your Game

"All you need are a pair of tennis shoes and motivation to change the course of your life."
— Heidi Bond[1]

Map your journey like a chess match, think ahead! It can be easy to get caught up with our next move. We know that we need to go to the gym at some point today. We know that we need to get in the kitchen and make our salad. Taking things one step at a time is going to be very helpful when you're getting started, but as we go along, we need to make sure that we are planning ahead. The more you can get in control of your destiny and all of the things that might happen which could affect it in the end, the better prepared you will be to handle whatever it is that might get thrown your way. Think of your next move. But then think of the move after that. It's simple, like the quote above. All we need to do is make sure that we have some solid shoes and a ton of motivation. It will make your journey easier, however, if you learn to plan ahead like you would in a chess match.

Be healthy in every aspect of your life, not just with what you are eating or how much you are exercising. Take care of yourself, starting with your mind. Be kind and careful with what you say to yourself. We will talk more about that later in the book as well. You need to take care of yourself in ways that don't just include this either. Take hot bubble baths, have a glass of wine while you binge your favorite show, buy a new dress for yourself right now, even though you might not be the ideal weight. I would tell myself that I didn't deserve new clothes all the time. I would always say that I shouldn't spend my money on bigger clothes when I could save it for a time when I had lost weight. But then I would go out to dinner with my husband, or an event for my children and have nothing cute to wear. I would just end up making myself feel bad because I didn't like the way I looked. You can't wait around for that confidence. Go out and get an outfit for yourself now that you like. Then when you lose the weight, you can keep it as a reminder and comparison for what your size used to be. I mean, don't go out and spend $100 on a dress you're only going to wear for a few months. But don't deprive yourself from shopping for your current size just because you don't think you will look good in it in your current self and size.

When it comes to taking care of yourself, I can't stress enough how much water you need to drink. On a daily basis, women need to drink at least two liters of water. This is the recommended amount. If you're wanting to lose weight, you really need to drink even more than that. I've had people tell me that they started drinking more water, but they still weren't seeing any of the effects, like clearer skin and a more regulated appetite. I would ask them how many glasses per day they were drinking and some would say at least one, maybe two (not including any coffee/tea/soda, and other beverages, simply water.) Then I would ask, "Ok, since you've made a conscious effort to drink more water, how many glasses are you drinking per day now?" They would say at least four, maybe five or six. That certainly wasn't enough to reach the daily-recommended amount! So even though they were drinking twice as much as they used to, it was still only half of what we actually need. Beyond that, as individuals that want to lose weight and get healthier, need to drink even more water. Eight glasses a day is what's recommended. So, you need to drink 10 or more to go above and beyond the recommendations. Invest in a glass or metal water bottle. I like metal ones because they tend to keep my water colder throughout the day. Room temperature water is actually the best for you, but I still like my icy cool glasses, which is better than not drinking water at all. Drink a glass of water as soon as you feel hungry. You will be amazed at how many times you were actually thirsty instead. Whenever I have an intense craving and I know I shouldn't give in, I will fill a glass of water and sip it for half an hour. Then, if the craving is still there, I might give in or at least eat a healthy snack, but most of the time, the water was enough to make that craving go away. We also have to make sure that when we're drinking water, we're actually sipping it and not chugging it. If you simply chug as much as possible at one time, you are just overloading your kidneys and that's not going to be helpful for your body's regulatory systems.

Everything that it is going to take for you to lose the weight already exists within you. When we really realize that, it can feel incredibly powerful. For so long we looked to the shelves at the supermarket, the many supplemental and vitamin stores, and the magazine rack filled with diet articles. While all these tools are helpful, the key to unlocking the powers of them all lies within you, in your own mind. That is a powerful feeling.

We all have energy inside of us; we all have power. It is what we decide to do with it that will be the most important. You can take that power and use it for evil. That power is your will to keep going, the motivation to continue on. You could take that energy and turn it inwards into something negative, making it easier to simply give up on your hopes and dreams and instead stay glued to the couch, watching more and more TV. Since it is such a strong force within our minds, if we're not careful with it, then we can end up using that power and turning it into something negative. Don't let this happen. Stay strong and keep pushing forward. The best way to do this is to plan ahead.

Saying No

Practice saying no! Whether you're saying no in the grocery store to the samples of cake and cookies, or no to having a second slice of pizza, this can be a powerful tool. We spent so much of our time saying yes that it became second nature. After a while, we didn't even realize that we were approving of our own bad habits. Many people's first word in their life is "no," and yet we still struggle to say it at the times when we need to use it the most. It's also a word that is common across many languages. It's almost as if it's a noise that we make, not even always a word. How many times do you think you've said it in your life? as we move forward, it's going to be a powerful tool that will help keep us on top of our game. Say "no" to others that might encourage you to want to be unhealthy. Maybe your family is asking to go to a certain restaurant where you know that all the menu items are deep-fried. It's OK to say no to this and find a place that works for both of you.

This involves saying no to ourselves as well. When we wake up in the morning, we can get the urge to just hit the snooze button one more time. Say "no" to the snooze button! Be strict with yourself like you would be with a child that you're trying to teach healthy lessons. Yes, sometimes it's not a big deal to have one cookie or to skip the gym just one day in a week. You're not going to fall off track from your diet because of this. However, we still need to learn how to say no to these situations, because if we don't then we can end up leading to other unhealthy habits. Think of saying "yes" as a gateway to other unhealthy behaviors. If you say "yes" once, then what's stopping you from saying it over and over again? Out of principle, say no when you can to try and keep things as focused as possible towards the goals that you want to achieve.

This was hard for me because I like to be kind to everyone, but we need to learn how to say "no" to others that are offering us unhealthy food. This would include my relatives, especially mom and grandma, always trying to get me to eat the brownies they just cooked. Or someone would text me and says, "let's go get pizza!" Even my husband would tell me I was being too strict and say, "just have a piece of cake." Every one of these people had only good intentions. They saw my resilient dedication as being too hard on myself, but it's what I needed to actually keep going. I don't hold anything against them, because I would tell other people the same thing if I saw how strong they were being. I encourage people to cheat now and then so that dieting doesn't have to be so challenging. However, I also know that one cookie might trigger me to eat ten more. Saying "no" to certain people is hard, but it's what we have to do to keep moving forward. No matter how sweet the person is and how much they show love through their food, your health is your top priority! When someone offers you food that can trigger you or you simply don't want to eat, say something like, "Thank you! This looks so amazing and you are so kind, but I am on a roll and I have lost five pounds! I have to keep up my momentum!" They will understand, and if they don't, well, that's on them. You can't beat yourself up if they take personal offense.

Never shame someone's food though. I've been around people dieting and they might get offered a piece of candy or a slice of pizza. Then they'll say to the person making the offer, "do you know how bad that is for you?" or "ew, that's so filled with sugar I'm not going to eat that." Never EVER make another person feel bad about what they're eating. Even if they offered you a deep-fried candy bar wrapped in bacon, they do not need to hear it from you that their food isn't good for them. Most people are usually aware on some level of the junk that they're eating, and if they're not, you don't need to shame them about it. Sometimes, it can be helpful to share the knowledge that they might not understand. For example, I had a friend that would often drink the pre-made fruit smoothies found in many grocery stores. She would have one every day and always wondered why she never lost weight. She would tell me "oh you should drink these they're so good!" Well, one day I went to get my own and looked at the nutrition facts seeing that they did include several fruits and veggies in them, but on top of that, a ton of sugar, almost as much as a bottled soda. I had to tell her, "these actually have a lot of sugar in them, and so it could be a factor in why you've had challenges losing weight. They taste SOOO good though, so I definitely understand the appeal!" Those might not have been my exact words, but I basically pointed out a fact, and also reminded her that her choice is totally valid, because it does taste good. I could have easily said, "these are so bad for you I would never drink something with so much sugar," but all that does is make her feel bad about herself. Just simply be polite when it comes to turning down food.

Sometimes this is just how we react because of the voice in our head that's been trained to think so negatively for so long. That voice in your head that's telling you to go to the drive thru or to skip the gym is so annoying! It sure is a loud mouth, isn't it? It's the first thing that pops into my head on a bad day, and it's the voice that can cause anxiety that keeps me up at night. Sometimes, that voice, the negative one that makes me feel bad about myself, is just so strong. It has become louder than our voices of encouragement at this point. That voice sure is loud when we don't need it, but where is it when we do? where's that voice encouraging us when we're running in the gym, or when we're doing our best to walk past the ice cream aisle? That voice sure is loud when we're feeling down about ourselves, but when we need a strong voice the most, it's nowhere to be found. Work on building your encouraging voice. This is going to best be done when we say "no" to our temptations.

Comparing Yourself

"The only person I am better than is the one I was yesterday." — Scott Deuty[2]

I absolutely love this quote. The only person that you should be in competition with is yourself. It can be very easy to start to compare yourself to others, and even form mini competitions in your mind. I would sometimes be competing with people that didn't even know they were part of a contest! In my head, I would try and compare myself to them and look for ways that

I was better, stronger, smarter, faster. The entire time, however, the other person didn't really care about any of this. It was a silly thing to do, but it's something that we all have to admit we've done before. The reason that we're so obsessed with comparing ourselves is firstly because we were taught to feel this way, especially women. We're told that if someone else is prettier, it means that you're not pretty at all. We're supposed to compare our bodies, even though we have completely different heights and structures. We also like to compare ourselves because it gives us a basis for structure and helps us define the things that seem more confusing. When you can think to yourself, "I'm a bad person, but not as bad as this other person I know," then it makes us feel better. But only momentarily. We have to learn to love ourselves and never worry about what another person is doing.

NEVER compare your weight loss success to your husband or your boyfriend! They will lose weight faster than you! I would do this a lot. When I would start to cook healthier or do something as simple as stop buying soda for the house, my husband would magically lose 15 pounds. He'd say something like, "look at my belt! I can move it to the smaller notch!" I'd smile and be happy that he managed to shed some weight, but he wasn't even trying. All that time I was busting my butt in the gym, skipping meals, and would still somehow manage to gain 5 pounds. It's just part of life! Men have a higher muscle to fat ratio and higher metabolisms! Unfortunately, their bodies are just more equipped to lose weight faster. It's frustrating, but it's something we have to accept. Comparison with men is only going to make us feel worse. You will get there! It might be harder, but you're only going to be stronger because of it. All of our bodies are different, and as someone that's overweight, we know that now. Even when we gain weight our bodies do it differently. Some people will gain all their weight in their thighs, others it will show up in their stomach. We have no control over where our bodies are going to store fat cells, so we can't compare our body at any size to someone else. Inside, the chemistry of our bodies is just as different. We also have to remember that we are going to pay a lot more attention to our own bodies than anyone else will to ours. We know that there's a little more cellulite on one leg versus the other, or that we have three rolls in our stomach compared to someone else's two. We know our worse angles, and the ones that make us look "slimmer." You can't compare yourself because other people are going to be looking at their own flaws and only focus on the issues they have with themselves.

We can't compare ourselves because we also don't know what the other person is going through. They might be thinking the same thing about themselves. As humans, we're naturally critical because it helps us to improve ourselves. If we never looked for our flaws, we would never find ways to grow and improve. However, we sometimes look way too closely at our flaws, and that's going to be just as damaging.

For every picture that someone posts online, remember that there might have been just as many bad pictures of their life that they would never share with you. I had a lot of issues online when I first started. I would look at my peer's social media pages and wonder what they had that I didn't that made them so happy. They would post pictures smiling, wearing bikinis, and cute selfies that they took out of nowhere. Their lives seemed perfect, and it made me feel worse about mine. It wasn't until I saw one of the people I followed online out in public. She had always posted cute pictures with her boyfriend, and they seemed like the perfect couple, like one that you would see advertising teeth-whitening strips together. They were picture perfect. However, they were also fighting, right in the middle of the grocery store. They didn't care who heard them and nothing about what was going on was cute. I realized then, that they're not going to post a picture about that. They were only showing me the greatest parts of their lives, the vacations, the happy days. They never posted the bad days or the ugly fights in the middle of the produce section. We have to remember this when we are looking at other's seemingly perfect lives online. Sometimes, the more confidence someone might seem to show in their pictures, the less they could have in their real life.

Planning Ahead

"Ambivalence is one of the biggest enemies of change. If you aren't sure that you really want

If you aren't 100% on board with something, then it's not going to help you find the success that you want. We have to make sure that we're going into this headstrong with a plan of action so that we don't get lost with our intentions. If we fall off track, then it can be so much harder to get back on. There have been a lot of diets that I would try where I didn't even fully feel like committing. It would just be the middle of March and I would think to myself, "I should probably diet since summer is coming up." Only, I was still suffering from the winter blues, so I didn't fully have the motivation level. I would just start the diet and hope that the rest would come along. You have to fully invest yourself and make sure that you're focusing on what's important. If you're ambivalent at all about this process, falling to plan and not doing much to ensure that you're ready for all obstacles ahead can be the reason that you don't find full success.

"Happiness is not the absence of problems, it is the ability to deal with them." — Steve Maraboli[4]

This is another incredible quote that I love. It's really just so true! We will always have problems, rich or poor, healthy or unhealthy, young and old. There are always going to be things that stress us out, that cause issues, which make us feel like we're going to just die.

There are moments of insecurity, uncertainty, discomfort, and frustration that will always come in and out of our lives. To think that we will ever reach a time where we have absolutely no problems is crazy. If we think that we will be truly happy when everything is resolved, then we are mistaking. We can't wait for happiness to come to us. We have to find it right now. Not having any problems isn't going to make you a happier person. Learning how to manage those problems and deal with them on an emotional level is exactly what you need to get to a place where you can live comfortably. It doesn't have to be so scary when it comes to accepting problems. Think about someone that's having a birthday party, and all the candles get lit to get blown out by the person whose birthday it is. As the cake gets carried out to them, the person trips and falls, causing the cake to go all over the place. This is a nightmare! Now no one gets cake and there's a big mess to clean up. But you know what? It's pretty funny. Yeah, the situation sucks, but as long as no one got hurt, it still causes everyone to laugh, and it's going to be a lot more memorable than any other birthday where there weren't issues. This is how we have to look at our life. When everything seems like a mess and things didn't go the way we planned, we just have to learn to laugh. When you can take on life as it is and see the bright side, funny side, or positive aspect from even the worst possible situation, then it will only make things easier for you moving forward.

Part of learning to not let the bad stuff affect you is going to be preparing for the worst. This isn't meant to inspire you to live with anxiety, but when we can assume the worst is going to happen, then what actually does happen, which is usually not that bad at all, won't seem so bad. Look for the things that are going to trigger you to want to go back to the way things used to be. When we are confronted with challenging times, then it makes us want to go back to old habits because it is reliable and dependable. If you experience a challenge, then it causes you to feel like things are out of control. You will look for that control by going back to the habits that once dominated your life.

Having a bad day at work and being too tired to cook when you get home is a huge trigger! I would sometimes just have a difficult day, whether I was tired and grumpy, and the regular tasks were harder, or even when I might have been in a good day but maybe a poor interaction with someone soured my mood. Either way, driving home, knowing that I would have to cook dinner made me feel even more stressed out. This would be when I would stop at a fast food join the most, not concerned that it would cause me to fall off track of my diet. I just wanted simplicity. I had gone through so much mental stimulation that day, negative too, that I just wanted something mindless so I could escape. While this isn't the best coping mechanism, it was what I had to do to make it through the day. we have to be prepared for these times because they will happen. To pretend like

100

you're going to have a perfect week isn't going to help you out in this struggle. Be realistic.

On your day off, have a meal prepared, freeze it if you need to for your rough days! Always have a backup meal ready for times that you aren't willing to cook. Even if it is a frozen meal that was pre-bought, which we don't recommend because they often have additives and fillers, it can still be better than loading up on greasy fast food. Think of this meal like a fire extinguisher ready in your freezer to put out the fire of your bad mood. Don't eat it just on any regular old day. only wait for when you're really struggling so that way you don't have to worry about falling off track when confronting a stressful time.

Have quick snacks that satisfy to grab! I make sure that I have protein bars, bags of nuts, and vegetable chips on hand for when I'm craving something. When my cabinets and drawers are empty, then this can be what really triggers me. Sometimes the cravings are so intense that I could cry, so I have to make sure that I have a backup. Even if I'm not craving that food that I kept, I will still eat it because it satisfies my appetite and then I'm not hungry at all for whatever it was that I was craving in the first place. You still want to manage how many snacks you're having, but being prepared is still better than not, which could lead to the desire to eat something that will ruin your diet.

Planning ahead is going to be a huge step in this monumental journey. If we pretend like we're going to be strong the entire time, then we're fooling ourselves. Another method I like to plan ahead is to buy the bad food I like to binge, but maybe a flavor I don't like. For example, I am a huge chocolate lover, especially ice cream. I could eat an entire pint of chocolate ice cream in one sitting. However, this can really set me back in a diet to keep it around my house. I struggle with being satisfied with just one serving, so I'll often overeat. To prevent this while still getting my ice cream fix, I'll get something that I don't like as much. I might get mint chocolate chip or peach, two kinds I still enjoy but not to the point that I want to binge them. I can have a scoop of them without having to eat the entire thing. When you're first starting out, try to do this. Rather than saying "I'm not going to buy any chips," maybe just try to buy the baked version or a cracker that you still enjoy, but don't like as much instead.

Moments of Stress

Have a healthy food snack cache in your desk, purse, car etc. to prepare for stress when you are apt to just grab anything. Stress can drive us to do crazy things. How many people have you heard say, "I want to pull out my hair!" when they are stressed? This didn't just come from nowhere. People will pull their hair out when stressed sometimes! It can cause stomachaches, headaches, back pain, jaw aches, and all sorts of other kinds of discomfort throughout your body. Stress can cause us to pick at our skin, fidget too much, and even fight with the people that we love the most. If you don't manage stress, it can lead to some serious times of emotional eating as well. We need to make sure that we are managing our stress so that we don't eat, but this is way easier said than done.

Stress can really drive us crazy and cause us to do things that we will regret. The worst part is, is that the things we do in an attempt to manage our stress can actually cause more issues in the end. Back to the discussion about eating fast food instead of going home and cooking, I would choose my favorite meal as a way to alleviate the stress from work. I could get a huge greasy burger and a large serving of fries, go home, eat that, but guess what? I was still stressed after! Not only did I have the residual stress of the workday to deal with, but I was also very mad at myself now for eating so much and falling off my diet track. The things that I tried to do to make my stress reduced just caused a lot more in the end.

When you are stressed out, your body releases cortisol, which can end up messing up bigger parts of your body. Stress isn't just all in your head. It can start there, but then you'll still end up feeling the effects elsewhere in your body if not properly managed. It's not just the way that we choose to feel and how we react. It's our body's natural response to stressful situations that cause a chemical reaction. Though we can control how we feel, it's not something that is easily done. We get better at it as time goes on, but there are still a ton of struggles that we have to go through that will help us build our stress management.

Stress can be blinding, so we have to prepare for these moments. This isn't just with food either. What other activates can you do that will help relieve stress? Exercise is a great way to get your blood pumping and mind thinking about something else. Start to exercise when you're in a good mood, however. If you say that you're only going to exercise after work, this will just cause more stress. Instead, maybe start working out every Saturday when you're in a good mood. Do it in the middle of the day if you want so that you can still sleep in. after consistently working out when you were in a good mood, it's going to be better to implement workouts in times of stress. Before you know it, you'll be pounding out workouts and relieving stress in the gym rather than in the kitchen.

Do your best to relieve stress throughout the day as well. Don't wait until your stress level is to the point where you're going to have an anxiety attack to do something about it. As soon as you feel the first moment of stress, breath and take a step back. Go outside and sit in nature if it helps you re-center your thoughts. Take a nap or a hot shower if you're stressed out at home. Make sure that you are stopping it as soon as you see it before you wait for it to explode and cause even more anxiety.

Travel

Traveling can be hard for many people. It's supposed to be all about fun. Traveling helps us learn more about ourselves and the world that we live in.

unfortunately, it can also cause us to do things that we wouldn't normally want to, such as eating an unhealthy meal. We might go on vacations, weekend trips, or even just a visit to a friend an hour away. Whatever the trip might be, we have to eat the entire time. It can be a lot harder to find an actual good meal that is totally healthy as well. When we're on vacation, we want to relax and have fun. This can mean that we might not be able to eat the tastier, unhealthier foods that everyone else we're on the trip is eating. While eating healthy and losing weight doesn't have to be a struggle, vacations are still all about indulging, and that means the food.

Decide before vacationing if you are going to cheat or if you are going to stay strong. Make a conscious decision based on your reality and your trip. Either way, your decision is fine, but you have to decide if you're going to stay rigid or not before going in. You can tell yourself, "We have to stay strong. We can't eat anything unhealthy this trip," but is that realistic? If you're going to Las Vegas where there's a buffet within every 50 feet, are you just setting yourself up for punishment by staying too strict? My mentality going into trips is to make healthier choices but to never stay too strict. Healthier choices also include making sure that you're being mentally healthy, and not being too hard on yourself.

When renting places, look for a hotel or Airbnb that has a fridge so that you can meal prep. This can allow you to bring healthy breakfasts like yogurt, eggs, and wheat toast. You can even have a healthy lunch too and eat a salad or some soup. Then, you can tell yourself that dinner you can get whatever you want. Another issue can be wanting to drink fancy cocktails filled with sugary juices while on vacation. I'll tell myself I can have one and then move onto red wine or even a light beer afterward. You can still have fun and enjoy your travels, it's just about making sure you're doing so in moderation and still being health-conscious.

Plan the places that you are going to eat ahead of time so you can see what their options might be. If you're trying to be strict, then you'll want to make sure you're choosing to go to places that will promote your diet, not potentially set it back. Vegetarian and vegan options, as well as things that are gluten free, are going to be helpful. These usually are prepared healthier and filled with food that is better for you overall. If you can make sure a restaurant has this menu, then you'll have good options for what to eat.

Bring a mini-cooler with healthy drinks in your car especially on long days of errand running/travel when you are most likely to justify a drive-thru trip. If your trip is short, even just a day, you should still be prepared. Remember not to beat yourself up. You can take a vacation from your diet. You just have to have a plan that will help you transition back into the real world when you're done. Going on a trip can be motivation for me as well. If I know I'm going to be on a sunny beach within a month, then I'll eat healthily and exercise and reward myself with the vacation. Not only will I look good in a bathing suit when the time comes, but I'll feel better about myself knowing I made the right choices. My reward isn't just the vacation, but also the fact that I allow myself to indulge in one meal a day while on the trip. I just have to make sure that while vacationing, I get in the mindset of knowing that it is ok to indulge and cheat and that I just have to make sure I'm dedicated when I go back to the real world.

Be Prepared When You Forget

Have a backup strategy when you forget all this! When you don't have food prepared, or a snack hidden, then what do you do? I get hungry in between breakfast and lunch sometimes, and at the end of the night when I'm just relaxing with my husband while watching TV, this is when I want to go to the cabinet and find something to binge. In order to prevent unhealthy habits at this time, I have to make sure that I'm preparing with a backup plan for my backup plan. This can include making sure that I have ingredients to whip up a snack, like granola bars or a yogurt parfait. I also might allow myself 1 strike in a week. This means that if it's Thursday and I managed to go Monday-Wednesday eating healthy, I can indulge in a meal one day, but I have to make sure I go right back to my diet the next moment.

Going to Restaurants

Going to restaurants would be the hardest part for me when it came to dieting. I would be doing great one week, but then out of the blue, I would get a text from a friend that would say something about taco Tuesday or boneless wings on thirsty Thursday. There were always moments that people would tempt me and saying no to that food sometimes meant saying no to a friend that I haven't seen in weeks. It's hard for me to turn down moments of hanging with my loved ones, so skipping the restaurant wasn't always the option. I would have a good week with my diet, but then eat a ton of junk at a restaurant, causing me to feel like I needed to give up. What I should have been doing was just ordering the healthier things on the menu.

Know your local drive-thru! There were a lot of moments when I was out with a friend or on a trip with family and they would all agree to just go to a drive-thru. On some days, especially with my two sons, we would just have to go for fast food because it was the quickest option for everyone. Avoiding restaurants like these are unavoidable. However, if we make ourselves aware of the healthier options on the menu, then we don't have to feel so bad about going. The majority of restaurants have healthy alternatives, especially nowadays.

Look at menus online before going to the restaurant. Then, you won't be ordering under pressure. Be aware of all the things that will ignite your cravings. I love nachos! I would die for nachos. Most restaurants have them in their appetizer section, loaded with a variety of greasy meats, cheeses, and other sauces that make this an unhealthy, dangerous choice. If I looked at a menu before I went, I would be aware that this trigger is present, making it easier to work through that craving and plan to order something healthier.

If you do want to cheat, enjoy it with someone else. It can be easier to make ourselves feel better about the choices we make when we do it with another person. Rather than ordering a burger with fries, ask if they would want to split that as well as a salad. Instead of eating that entire unhealthy meal, you're eating less of it and sharing the calories with someone else. It allows you to eat the food you crave without eating the entire portion, which might inflate your weight.

Eat before you go out as well so that you can only eat a small amount. If I knew I was going to a tasty dinner, I would sometimes starve myself all day just to build the anticipation. All this would do is cause me to overeat and order way more than I needed. Instead, now, I make sure to drink a huge glass of water and have at least a snack, maybe even a salad. Always order a salad with your dinner as well if it doesn't already come with one on the menu. Make sure you eat the entire thing to fill yourself up before the meal gets there. Then, you can easily just eat a smaller amount of that food.

Before you start eating, cut it in half. Especially in the U.S., portion sizes can be more damaging than the nutritional value of the actual food. Whatever it is that you ordered, whether it's a plate of pasta or an entire sandwich, split it right down the middle. Then you can eat half and take the other half home. You can see before you start eating how much food there is so that you don't get ahead of yourself and eat a huge amount. I would often go to restaurants and eat to the point where I was stuffed, but there was still some left on my plate. It wouldn't be enough to justify taking home, but it was still a significant amount that I wouldn't want to waste, especially if it were a more expensive meal, so I would eat it even though I was beyond full. If you separate a portion to take home before you start eating, then you can be assured that you won't have to worry about overeating.

Suggest restaurants that you don't even like as much if you have to. This way, you won't be as tempted to eat your entire meal. If a friend says, "let's go to dinner! I was thinking either this restaurant or this one." And you hate the second one, pick that. You will be less likely to binge, and you know that the other person will like it since they suggested the restaurant in the first place.

Parties

Parties can be very challenging, especially if we're drinking alcohol. There are so many empty calories in all of these drinks and beer and wine can have a huge amount of sugar even though they don't taste as sweet. Make sure that you are focusing on your alcohol content just as much as you are the food that you're choosing to eat. Drink in moderation. The less we drink, the higher our tolerance is, so the less we have to drink later on.

Eat healthy BEFORE going to the party so you won't eat as much at the party. If you know that the party you're going to is going to have a long table full of different snacks, then fill yourself up so that you're not as tempted to keep snacking. Instead of grabbing a spoonful of dip and a handful of mini hot dogs at the party, just make a small platter. Let yourself take a sample, have one bite, and just a taste rather than creating a heavy plate that looks like you came from a buffet.

Don't eat snacks. If there's a bowl of chips on the table, just say NO. I would often find myself eating an entire bowl of pretzels while having conversations without even realize it! Now I know how dangerous this can be, so I'll sit somewhere far from any food, or I'll move the bowl in front of me towards my sons and husband so that they can eat the snacks to resist my temptation.

Decide before going if you are going to tell others or not about your dieting. Telling other people can help encourage you because they might be helpful, telling you not to eat certain foods and avoid asking. In the beginning for me, however, I was afraid to tell others because I didn't want them to judge me. If I failed my diet again, I would look so silly. IT's definitely not the truth, but it's how I felt. It's up to you to determine if telling others about your diet is going to hurt or help you.

You can also use the party as a chance to actually cheat. Maybe you know that there's a birthday party on Friday. Tell yourself all week that you can go crazy at this party, eating as much cheese pizza and cake as you want, but only if you succeed the rest of the week. This would usually give me encouragement to stick to a diet, and then when the party got there, I would still feel encouraged from accomplishing my goals, leading to me only wanting to have a few slices of pizza anyway.

Your Hormones

For biological females that experience their menstrual cycles, this can be a very challenging part of your journey that could cause you to make some unhealthy decisions. Not only are our stress levels higher, but our cravings seem more intense as well.

When your monthly hormones kick in, allow yourself a couple squares of low sugar dark chocolate a day until cravings subside. Don't try to torture yourself when you're already in pain and feeling miserable. If you do, then it can become a lot harder to stick to your diet. Instead, be realistic and understand that you're

112

going through a tough time when on your period and give yourself a chance to have some chocolate.

This helps with sweets and carb cravings. Prepare yourself mentally to gain fluid weight during your period! I make sure to not weigh myself at all, measure my waist, or wear anything too tight while on my period because I know I'll feel bloated. Trying to fit into my skinny jeans doesn't do me any good while on my period because I just feel like I've gained weight. I know now that sweats or at least leggings are going to be the best option.

For me, the second and third days of my period are the hardest. The first isn't great but I make it through. Then on the second and third, however, I sometimes feel like if I don't get some chocolate or red meat that I'm going to murder someone.

Our bodies will be craving iron because of blood loss, so it is important that you are replenishing that. Plan meals around red meats this week, but make sure they are still healthier options. Allow yourself to be a little grumpy and know that it's just your hormones. Don't make any decisions about your diet now either. Just do your best to stick to your regimen.

Weighing Yourself

The scale can be a very dangerous site for many people going through a weight loss journey. The numbers fluctuate so much, and we can end up staring at those three little symbols more than we pay attention to our own bodies. People might think that they're still overweight just because they don't weight as little as a friend, disregarding what their bodies even look like. You should try to avoid the scale as much as possible and only weight yourself throughout longer periods of time.

Weigh yourself at the same time. Our bodies will change a lot throughout the day, so if you are inconsistent with time, that can affect your results. Don't weigh daily! Please, please, please do not weigh yourself every day or every other day. I would say once a week is the maximum that you should be.

Anything more than that will just cause you to be emotional. One day you might weight 198, the next day 203, and that can cause you to feel terrible about yourself. You might go off track with your diet even though if you had weight yourself the third day, you'd weight 197. Our weight fluctuates depending on what we eat, our bowel movements, and the water that we're retaining.

Don't let this affect you negatively! Sometimes we have to gain a little more weight before we lose it. Remember that your weight loss isn't going to be consistent. You are going to lose a lot more in the beginning than you will later on. You might lose 20 pounds in a month, but the next month only 10. This is because when we first start off, we lose a lot of water weight. As time goes on, you're going to lose weight less consistently, but don't let this discourage you. It is part of life!

1) Bond, H. (2016). <u>Who's the new kid?</u>
2) Deuty, S. (2019). <u>Secrets of an Over 50 Former Fat Man.</u>
3) Spangle, L. (2007). <u>100 Days of Weight Loss: The Secret to Being Successful on Any Diet</u>
4) Maraboli, S. (2014). <u>Life, the truth, & being free.</u>

Chapter 4 – Get Back Up!

"If I'm going to have hope, I'm going to have to learn to endure disappointment." — Sharon Weil[1]

Throughout the book so far, we've given you the strategies needed to keep you prepared so that you don't fall off track. If you don't want to make a mistake, it's important to prepare for that to happen. What we have to realize is that mistakes are inevitable, so now that we know what to do to prevent them as much as possible, we need to now go over what to do when you do make that mistake. You might fall off track for the first ten times, but what matters most is that you still get up the eleventh time. Every time you make a mistake or do something you regret, it is over an instance that has ended. We always have the biggest feelings of remorse for things that are in the past, what can no longer be controlled.

After you "mess up" then you have to get back on your feet. Sometimes we don't want to give second chances to people that have made mistakes in the past, but we don't have the option of cutting ourselves out of our lives. For that reason, we tend to punish ourselves a lot harder than we do other people. If someone messed up and hurt us through a certain mistake they made, then it can be easy to say that we're going to just distance ourselves and spend some time apart while we recover from their "mess-up." However, we can't really avoid ourselves, so we have to face these issues head on and come up with a proper solution.

Failing can just make success feel so much better. If you never failed once in your life and succeeded with everything that you ever tried, then success would be natural. It wouldn't feel as good to you because it's what you expect. However, if we experiencing failing a few times, when we finally get to appreciate all the greatness that comes along with finally achieving the goals we've been wanting. It's not like we should intentionally fail for this reason, however, when you made it to the end, look back on your life to see all the mistakes you've made. All those times you felt like a failure have just become learning lessons. There is such a stigma around failure that we fear it to the point that it stops us from even trying something new in the first place. We can't allow this mentality to consume our lives. We have to start now working towards a better future where we accept that failure is inevitable.

This is a great way to look at all of our past mistakes as well. Everything you've done in this life has led you to this moment. I made some mistakes, not related to my weight, in my childhood, teen years, early adulthood, and so on. If I hadn't made one mistake, it might have led me down another path. Who knows, I might have made a decision that changed my life so drastically that I never would have met my husband. If that hadn't happened, I wouldn't have my beautiful children now, and I can't imagine a life like that. Though I have my regrets, I'm grateful for everything that I've been through, good and bad, because it made me who I am today.

There is surely something in your life right now that you are proud of. Whether it's your job, where you live, your boyfriend, your group of friends, or anything else, you have to have at least one thing that you're proud of. If you hadn't made every decision that you have in your life, including the choices you might have made regarding your diet choices, then you wouldn't be the person you are now, with the things in your life that made you proud. If you honestly can say that you're not proud of anything, that nothing in your life has brought you joy, well then, you only have upwards to go. It might feel like everything is terrible, and there's a chance that you're struggling to find anything that makes you happy. But even this challenging time is still a learning lesson. You will have success one day, and then you can look back on this time when you felt no joy for anything and use that pain to remind you to keep going forward. Sometimes we have to hit bottom so that we have a good solid ground to push off from.

How You are Reacting

"Excuses don't kill the fat, exercises do." — Amit Kalantri[2]

I can think of a million excuses for why I might want to eat a certain food, skip my exercise, or just quit my diet altogether. The unfortunate thing about excuses is that they are very easy to find. Sometimes my excuse for eating a candy bar was that I didn't want it to go to waste. Guess what? Eating it is still wasteful when you're on a diet! I eat it, I don't get hardly any nutrients out of it, and then I poop it out. It becomes waste anyway, just in a different way! This is no excuse. The more excuses we make, the more detached from the truth we are.

We make excuses because it's easier than having to confront the truth and admit that we are actually responsible for the mishap.

You are not wrong for having a slip-up. You would be wrong if you let this be the determining factor for if you are going to fail. When you fail, you have two options. You can either let it consume you and take over your life, or you can let it be a reminder that you are human, and you just have to be a little stronger next time. Let's think about a common scenario I would find myself in, and that my clients have discussed as well. You start a diet and it goes great for the first, let's say, four days. Then, on day five, you get home and your friend/spouse/roommate has ordered a pizza and it's sitting on the counter. They tell you to grab a slice and you think right away that you shouldn't be eating that. The gooey cheese is calling your name, and you could smell it from the hallway as you walked into the kitchen. It's irresistible, so you decide to take a slice, even though it can throw your diet off-track, especially if you're doing a keto diet. Then on day six, you think to yourself, what's the point of going on with my diet? I've already ruined it.

This kind of mentality is toxic! Yes, you messed up. You did something you shouldn't have. But that's no reason to throw in the towel. In a week, month, a year, five years, that one slice of pizza, or however many you ate, will have no significance to you if you decide to forget about it and carry on. After six months of dieting, you won't even remember that dumb piece of pizza! However, if you let that be your excuse for quitting the diet, then it will be significant. In a month, then you won't have lost the weight you could have if you had stuck with the diet in the first place. Make sure you always choose to just dust yourself off and get back up.

Think of the most inspirational person you can. If they failed, what would you do? It took thousands of tries to try and create the light bulb. If the inventors of all the greatest things in our lives had given up after the first, fifth, tenth, or even hundredth time they tried and failed, how different would our lives look? What matters is never really that you had a slip-up. What the issue will be is whether or not you are handling that in a healthy way.

You will mess up, you are human, and it is how you react to it that matters! Reactions are what are always important in all scenarios as well. If someone makes you mad, it's not your fault for getting mad. However, you can choose to keep your cool, say something about it and move on. Or, you can choose to throw a fit, yell, and punch the wall. We have to be aware of our reactions and how they might be affecting us so that we can move in a direction of success.

We can become so scared of failing that we never try in the first place. There can be comfortableness felt within consistent failing. It is a cycle that can almost become a habit. You try, you mess up, and you quit. You decide to try again, but then there's a mess up, and then you quit again. This can happen over and over again until it's the only behavior that we're expecting from ourselves. Don't let this become your normal. If this is the cycle that you're already in, then it's time to break it!

Speak to Yourself Like You Would a Friend

From here on out, never say anything to yourself that you wouldn't say to a friend. I've said such terrible things to myself that if I ever said anything like that to another person, I would've gotten slapped! I've looked in the mirror and told myself that my body was disgusting, hideous, embarrassing, and shameful. I've cried in the dressing room too many times over how much I absolutely hated my body. However, I've never looked at a friend with such hate. Even if someone is twice my size, I would never in a million years look at them and think that they were disgusting. So why, then, was it so OK for me to say these kinds of things to myself?

Would you call your dog a failure? Your little sister, cousin, or other small child? Anytime you say something terrible to yourself, make sure you repeat it out loud. It can be easy to let thoughts slip into our head. When you are forced to say it out loud, then you might realize just how terrible of a thing it really was to say. This can help you overcome these harmful statements.

That voice in your head isn't always right. It's strange how easily our mind can play tricks on us. You might say something and think that it's true just because it was the thought that popped into your head. We are constantly having conversations with ourselves in our head. We talk to ourselves more than other people! For this reason, we have to be our own best friend. A friendship consists of love and compassion, so you need to start showing that to yourself. There is nothing that's going to be helpful from a bad attitude and making yourself feel better. Bullying yourself is only going to make you feel worse. That angry voice comes from a place of pain as well. It didn't just form overnight. It took a while to get that angry voice buzzing in your head, so it might take a while to get it to dissolve as well.

The first thing we think is what we were taught. Whether it's a thought you have when you see yourself or someone else, that first thing you think is what your brain was conditioned to create. The second thing shows our true character. What you think after that, how you might remedy what you say next, that is what matters most. Sometimes, I'm not going to lie, I might be talking to someone and the other person says something pretty ignorant. In my head I think, "they're so dumb." This is just what I was taught, however. I was told growing up through peers and society that a person that says something stupid is simply a stupid person. However, my second thought will be, "they're not dumb, they just didn't know any better about that one thing they were told." Unfortunately, a lot of people will only have that first voice articulated, and it will be a lot louder than the other voices. We have to make sure that we are training that second voice and making it as loud, in fact, louder, then the first thought that pops into our head.

When you say to yourself, "what's wrong with you that you can't do this," or something along those lines, don't give into that. There's going to be no benefit from being that hard on yourself. That voice that breaks us down is pretty strong and thinks it knows it all. Where is that voice, then, when we need it the most?

Have a Mess Up Strategy

Each time you mess up, evaluate that. What triggered it? Sometimes nothing at all, and that's completely fine. It can sometimes be a natural reaction to self-sabotage or just simply mess up because we get scared, or because that's what's expected. We have to make sure that we are being mindful of this, however, and always try to evaluate what exactly it was that led us to think a certain way or make a certain decision.

If you have to, write a contract to yourself. This would be something that you can look at and go back to when you do mess up and remind yourself that it is OK and perfectly acceptable to make mistakes. Create this contract when you are in a good mood and feeling motivated. Then, when you mess up, you can go back to it and realize that you have to follow what you originally said if you want to find any success at all. It might include something like this:

"I will allow myself one meal to go crazy this week on then I will be back on track. I will have a recovery day with extra water. I will NOT beat myself up psychologically because this is NORMAL behavior, it only becomes abnormal and destructive if I wallow in negativity and continue to stay out of control and overindulge."

Whatever it might be, prepare to fail just as you are preparing to become motivated. You know what? You might not fail. You might hit it off perfectly this time around. However, we can't expect this. It isn't that we have low standards, it's just that we're being realistic. Low standards would be us laughing at ourselves for even trying in the first place. Always prepare to fail, no matter how discouraging that might sound. This is because failure is such a stigma, but a lot more people fail than succeed, so it's completely normal behavior. If we consistently make strategies to pull us out of moments that we "fail," then it will become a lot less frequent that we have mess-up moments.

We have to change our perspective on failing. When you can accept it as part of your life and embrace the lessons that can come along with failing, then you will feel much better about the situation in the end.

Never Make Yourself Feel Guilty

Sometimes, we might think that punishing ourselves is the way to elicit positive change. If a dog pees in the house, you might crate it as punishment. If your child hits their sibling, then you might put them in time-out. Punishment shouldn't be for ourselves just because we wanted to eat something tasty! We can't be the punisher and the punished at the same time. This is just going to cause more issues in the end.

How can you expect positive outcomes based in negativity? When you're in a terrible mood, feeling really low about yourself, and wanting to just give it all up, how can you expect to inspire positivity with this outlook? Instead of trying to get something good to happen out of a negative mood, we have to first focus all of our attention on simply changing our mood from one of anger to one of happiness.

Negative reinforcement never works. If you are trying to teach a dog to sit, then you will give them a treat after every time they sit. You wouldn't punish them every time that they don't sit! The more love and compassion we can give ourselves, the happier we will be. The happier we are, the easier it will be to make positive decisions. The easier that is, the more likely we will be to actually find success.

1) Weil, S. (2018). <u>Changeability</u>.
2) Kalantri, A. (2019). <u>Wealth of Words.</u>

Chapter 5 – A Lifelong Journey

"The man who moves a mountain begins by carrying away small stones." — Confucius[1]

I love this quote! When we think about having to do something successful, we often get caught up with the idea that we have to do things all at once. I had so many clients that were upset they didn't lose 50 pounds in the first month of their diet. That is not only unhealthy but pretty much impossible. Our bodies don't work that quickly! It took a long time to put all that extra weight on your body, so it's going to take a while to get it off as well. This is a marathon, not a race. You have to pace yourself. If you're casually jogging instead of sprinting, then you're going to have a much lower chance of tripping and falling.

It is going to take just as long to change to a positive lifestyle as it took to get into a negative one. Unfortunately, we conditioned ourselves to think in a certain negative way. Too often, we felt like we were not working toward our "success" or whatever we had defined it as, if we couldn't measure it in large tangible amounts. We have to start to look at the smaller things in life that can lead to success. Not everything has to be so big, so overdone. Instead, we can simply look at our jeans being a little loose on us as a massive milestone, rather than expecting to be able to fit into a much tinier size right away. Learn to take things in smaller amounts and after a while, you will be able to see the bigger picture.

We have to focus on methods that we can measure our success. Often, people will do this with numbers. They will hop on a scale, pull out a tape measure for their waste, or look at how quickly they might have been able to lose a certain amount of weight. None of this matters! You have to instead focus on the little milestones and how you feel overall. Sometimes, we measure success too much in ways that we think we can quantify. Everyone's journey will look different, and that includes the successes we manage to make along the way.

You did your best, that's something that should be rewarded. If you can say that you honestly tried, then you should feel proud. You might not have gotten exactly what you wanted out of a certain situation, but you should still feel incredibly proud that you attempted something without giving up. As you move along your journey, your successes can get a bit easier to measure, and you will also have larger goals. That is fine though because you will have the tools needed to achieve those more challenging goals.

There are days I've woken up and thought, I'm going to run an entire mile right now. But then I would get out of bed and feel tired, not wanting to go on a run at all. Even though I had no desire to run, I would at least put my workout gear on and try. I think about how I would want to be able to sprint and get it over with, but I was really lacking the motivation. Some days, I pushed through and managed to run the entire mile, maybe even more. Other days, I would have to just give up and turn back home. Some days I got more success than others, and there were times when I would go beyond what I expected to achieve. What mattered most at the end of the day was that I had still gotten myself up and to a place where I was willing to try and finish, no matter how scary that might have been.

"Doing things faster is doing things slower." — Martin Berkhan[2]

Finding Support Groups

Asking for help can be scary, but sometimes, it's exactly what we need to find the right kind of motivation. Join a Facebook support group or local support group that is positive and everyone is on a similar journey. You can easily find these types of groups, you just have to be willing and open to accepting that you might need others to do this. You can really learn a lot from yourself and the journeys you go through, but you can learn so much more from other people. Some individuals will simply be better at articulating a certain thought or feeling than you would, so it's important that you are doing your best to be open to new people and finding help from others.

We have so many tools already in ourselves needed to find success. Luckily, other people have already discovered those, so it can help to quicken the process of self-discovery. Talking to someone else can sometimes be enough to help you find what you need.

We think all day, constant thoughts passing through our heads. It's only when we say some of them out loud that we can truly understand what they mean. If you're able to talk to someone, it can help you work out the feelings that you have so that you can better understand what it is that they might exactly mean.

Asking for help can be scary. It might mean admitting that you are not as strong as you think you are. We like to think that we can do it all on our own, that we're the ones in charge of our destiny. What we have to remember, however, is that we are also in charge of where we might find help and when.

We can't measure strength by what we're capable of doing ourselves. We can measure strength by how accepting we are of reality, and how much love we have for ourselves. Imagine that there's a log in the middle of the road blocking traffic. If you got out of the car and were trying to pick it up yourself, turning down everyone else that tried to help, would this make you look strong? No! In fact, it would make you seem weaker to others that you're not willing to enlist in their help. What would make you look strong is if you were to assign roles to other people, telling a few people to stand at the end of one log, a few at the other, and then guide everyone to lift at the same time and move it together. Sometimes, our biggest strength is recognizing that we need the help of others. Asking for help is just another tool that will carry you further in this crazy journey.

Start Your Own Group

Start your own group! If you're having trouble finding one in your area, or simply if you want to create another type of group, you can do this on your own! You could hold meetings at your home, on Facebook, or talk to other public spaces to see about renting or borrowing the area for your meeting. A great way to help others and heighten your level of accountability. If you take responsibility for the inspiration of others, it can help to keep yourself motivated. You will want to give up sometimes, but then you'll remember that others are depending on you, looking up to you, and coming to you for advice and support. This will help remind you that you can not only let yourself down, but you can't let down all the others that are there to help you.

Remember that you are not in control of anyone and that trying to do this too early can be triggering. If you are starting your journey now, then wait at least a year before you try to become accountable for helping others. Not only do you want to make sure you've worked out all the kinks in your recovery plan and really realized all the things that matter most, but you will make sure that you're not putting too much pressure on yourself. You have to go at it a little slower at first, and then as time goes on you can start to reach out and help others.

Sometimes it is a lot easier to help other people than it is ourselves, so don't let this become a distraction. I could sit and talk to my patients all day about what they need to do to change. I can tell them all the things they're doing wrong and give them advice on how they need to better their lives. Unfortunately, when it comes to managing my own weight, it's a lot more challenging. Especially in the beginning, I would latch onto other people's problems and try to take accountability for those before addressing my own issues. This was just a way to distract myself and make me feel like I accomplished something. Don't get me wrong, helping people is very important it is something that we should strive to do. however, if we focus solely on helping each other and never ourselves, then it's only going to only hurt us in the long run.

Setting Goals

When it comes to your weight loss journey, you have to make sure that you are setting the right goals. Don't measure progress with a scale! It can be very easy to get into a mentality where you are only tracking your progress by how much weight you've lost and how small your waist is. We need to measure our success by how good we feel! Be mindful of how you feel now and what might be caused by your weight. I always had a lot of back pain, and my knees were very sore from doing the bare minimum before my weight loss. As I got in shape, I started to realize that my back didn't hurt at all. I didn't care that I was 30 pounds down, I cared that I could go for a run without coming home and feeling my knees throb for the next four hours.

Goals should be set no matter what, even if you are trying to casually lose weight. That is what's going to help you stay on track. Smaller goals are just as important. Sure, you might want to lose 100 pounds. First, however, make it a goal to lose five pounds. When you've reached that goal, make your next one to lose 10 more pounds, then 20 the next time. after that, you've reached 35 pounds down, so now your goal can be to double that. Once that goal has been achieved, then you can make it your goal to lose 100 pounds. By doing these smaller goals, it gets a lot easier to see our success. If your goal is to just lose 100 pounds, then it will take so long for you to achieve a goal and feel good about yourself. After six months, if you had set smaller goals, then you likely would have hit that 35-pound mark, and you'd be feeling great. However, if you didn't set those smaller goals, after six months you'd barely be halfway there, so you might feel like giving up because progress still seems so far away.

Think of your success like a bridge over water. A bridge goes from one point to the next. The basic foundations exist on each point on the land. However, there are a lot of much smaller foundational structures that exist in between those points. If it was just across one point to the other, then it would collapse in the middle. Instead, bridges have larger support beams throughout the entire thing to keep it solid. Think of your journey like the bridge. Each of those smaller foundational structures along the way is the goal that is going to help you build a really solid bridge between who you used to be and the person that you're going to become.

Rewards Over Punishments

Sometimes I would have moments where I punished myself, and my patients would punish themselves as well. I've spoken to a lot of people that would eat a ton of junk food, only to starve themselves for the next three days as a form of punishment. There were many individuals that would go as far as making themselves throw up as well. They thought that if they punished themselves, then they would be more successful in the end.

Here's the thing about punishments: they're meant to teach a lesson. When you were a child and you stole a toy, you would get punished by your parent as a way to teach you that stealing is not acceptable. Our parents knew that what we did is wrong, so they could come up with an appropriate punishment. As children, we didn't know any better, but we learned from our parents. If you are punishing yourself, then you are already aware of the consequence! When you come up with the terms of your punishment, it's to teach a certain lesson, only, you already know the point of the lesson, which is why you're trying to enforce it. Why then, would we punish ourselves if we already know the consequences of our actions?

It can be easy to get into a mentality of sacrificing something for the sake of learning a lesson. We can't punish ourselves.

Instead, we have to deal with the consequences and become aware of them. I noticed for my patients that it was sometimes easier for them to simply punish themselves rather than confronting the root issue that was actually wrong in the first place.

Positive reinforcement is going to be more helpful. Don't wait until you've failed to take action. Give yourself positive reinforcement as often as possible. This is what I was talking about when it comes to working hard all week only to have a nice, unhealthy meal on the weekend as a reward. We need to give ourselves as much compassion as possible so that we can keep succeeding. Don't beat yourself up. Brush your shoulders off and instead move forward. Always reward yourself. Put much more of an emphasis on reward than punishment.

Give Yourself Permission

We have to start to learn how to give ourselves permission to do different things. Allow yourself to have a snack, let yourself eat an extra cookie. Whatever it might be, you have to learn how to say that it is "ok" to do certain things.

Imagine right now that you are in charge of watching a small child. You are in that child's home, and there's a very expensive looking vase on a shelf. You tell the child, "whatever you do, DO NOT touch that vase." What do you think the child will do immediately as soon as you leave the room? They're likely going to touch that vase.

If you didn't point out that expensive vase, the child might have never noticed it. By building their curiosity, you've led them to do the one thing they shouldn't. If you hadn't said anything at all, they probably wouldn't really care. If you said, "you can touch that vase if you want," they might have still ignored you and found something else interesting to touch. This isn't true for all kids, but it's the way that we can look at how making things off limit in our own minds can only lead to more curiosity down the road.

When we say, "this is the last piece of pizza I'll have for months," then immediately we want more pizza. When we say, "no more fast food," then all we can do is think about the greasy burger from our favorite drive-thru. If you give yourself absolutes, then you can cause stress, which can lead to the feeling of wanting to eat even more.

Tell yourself that you can eat whatever you want. Give yourself permission to have cheat days, to binge eat, to skip exercises, and you'll realize that the desire to do this is much less. Say, "you can eat all the candy in the kitchen, and you can order a pizza just for yourself if you want." But you also have to remind yourself of the consequences. When we do this, we will be much more likely to make the right decision rather than one based on anxiety and curiosity.

When we remove something from our lives that gave us meaning, then it can cause panic. It's a natural instinct to become scared or upset if something with meaning is being taken from us. Don't give yourself such strict restrictions with what you're allowed to do, and you will find that it's much easier to stick to a healthy diet.

Always Look to the Root

The most important thing you are going to have to do throughout this journey is to challenge your thoughts. Each and every thought that passes through your mind is one that you need to question. Every time you let something pop into your head, you have to ask where it came from and how it got there in the first place. Was it something that you said to yourself? Maybe it's the hurtful words of the bullies on the playground. Perhaps the words you're hearing came directly from your own parents. No matter where it came from, we have to question why we think a certain way so that we can understand our root issues.

Ask yourself "why" after every mean thing you say to yourself. When I look in the mirror and think, "gosh I look gross today," I question why I think that. I'll say, "well, my hair is frizzy, my stomach is bloated, and I'm breaking out." Then I ask, "why does that make you gross?" I keep asking why until I realize that the thoughts I'm having aren't legitimate, and I need to focus my energy on thinking other things.

When we really dig deep to the root, we can see where it originated. It can be hard. It's not always easy to do this. It sometimes means that we will have to work through our most negative thoughts that are engrained deeply into our minds. Keep asking yourself "why" like a two-year-old would as they're discovering all the complexities of life.

A lot of this might mean confronting childhood trauma. You might find that the hurtful words you tell yourself came from an abusive parent, or maybe a long-term bully. You have to be ready to challenge these thoughts no matter how painful they might be. If it is something that becomes too challenging for you, you might find more help from talking this out with a therapist or other mental health professional.

By the time you work out your issues, you might not even have that craving, or desire to skip the gym anymore. You might have worked through those feelings of wanting to just stay home and instead created the motivation to keep going and work through the issues.

Binge Eating

Binge eating is an eating disorder that a lot of my patients struggled with. This involves eating far beyond the amount of food that is needed to make you less hungry. Those that binge eat won't just eat a large bowl of ice cream. They will eat an entire carton to the point that they feel sick. Binge eating isn't enjoyable. Those that do it don't eat mindfully, thinking about how good it tastes. They are usually eating to fill an emotional void that they haven't fully recognized.

This is caused by the desire to take control over your life, but it ends up happening in the wrong way. Therapy can be very helpful for this. If you think that you might have a binge eating disorder, then you might want to talk to a professional to see what the best method of treatment is.

Binge eating is more than just food. There are deep-rooted emotional issues that can lead to this type of behavior. Being mindful of what you are eating and why you are having the desire to binge is going to be crucial in overcoming this battle. Just like why we might skip diets, looking at why we binge eat will be very important in overcoming any of your inner battles.

1) Confucius., & Waley, A. (2000). The Analects.
2) Berkhan, M. (2018). The Leangains Method.

Chapter 6 – Positive Relationships

"Words are easy, like the wind; Faithful friends are hard to find." — William Shakespeare[1]

There are so many people in the world that we don't have to worry about a shortage of bodies to surround us. What we do have to be concerned with, however, is how many of those people are actual faithful friends that we can trust to stand by us even in the most challenging of times. Surround yourself with people making largely positive choices in their lives, you become who you hang around. If at the moment all of your friends are participating in bad behaviors that keep them as consistently unhealthy individuals, then we won't' be able to fully find the help that we need to make it through this challenging journey. This doesn't mean that right now, you have to cut out everyone in your life that isn't healthy. We do, however, have to make sure that we are seeking out a healthy support system filled with people that are going to help drive us in a direction to making positive decisions for ourselves. Distance yourself from people with the victim/excuse driven mentality. This can be very contagious! Excuses are likely what got you here in the first place. If only people that keep making excuses for their own behavior surround you, then that kind of thinking is going to get into your head and affect your varying perspectives. You can easily start to feel as though this is a way of life and how you should be feeling. When you have so many people in your life that think that they aren't at fault and don't accept responsibility for their actions, then it can lead to the entire group thinking that, therefore everyone's excuses mentality becoming validated. If someone else is telling you that what you're doing or thinking is right, no matter how healthy or unhealthy it is, then you will think that you are right. This can lead to a feeling of solidifying those unhealthy emotions that got you there in the first place.

Seek out the friends at the gym that are making progress and have found the mental groove of success! Just like how a negative mindset might end up seeping into your thought process, a positive one can just as easily. Success is contagious too! If you are with others that are going to consistently encourage you, then it's only going to make that journey easier in the end. You have to find people that are going through the same things as you and understand what it's like to experience the struggles that you have. If we do this, then we can better make sure that we are finding the support needed to really make it through this journey.

Anyone that tries to bring you down has their own problems. I'll never understand a person that thinks they should tell someone else how to live their life by belittling them and mocking their behavior. I had a coworker one-time laugh at me because I took the bun off my burger and simply ate the patty and veggies after a work BBQ. "Just eat the damn burger!" She said laughing. Sure, it was a silly sight to see someone eating a burger with a fork and knife. But I was having a great day and feeling really good about myself. I enjoyed the BBQ without having to break my diet, and that motivated me to keep going the rest of the week. Seeing her laugh and roll her eyes hurt. By her making me feel like my choice to eat that burger the way I was is silly made me feel like every other part of my struggle was meaningless as well.

People like to point out your flaws so that they don't have to look at their own. That woman that made fun of me likely had her own body issues. She might not have even realized she was hurting me, but that doesn't make it any better. The only reason that another person would feel the need to point out your flaws and the things that you do that are embarrassing is usually because they don't want to have to think about the issues that they have that bother themselves. This is why it can become easier to not worry when someone is judging you. The more I can focus on myself and not worry what other people think, the easier it will be to stay confident in my regimen and stick to a plan that works.

Losing weight can sometimes mean overcoming everything that others have said to you. I had a ton of patients who had parents that were very hard on them, sometimes even blatantly calling them "fat." This kind of talk is disgusting, especially coming from a parent. It's important that parents are worrisome over their children's health but telling a 12year-old girl that she's huge or fat isn't going to make her want to eat a salad. Instead, she'll probably feel bad about herself to the point that she might binge eat.

> *"People who have character, follow through. They don't lie to themselves or anyone else. They don't start something, then give up because it is "hard." People of character set a goal and stick to it."* — Nancy Mure[2]

How You Were Raised Counts

> *"People are always blaming their circumstances for what they are. I don't believe in circumstances. The people who get on in this world are the people who get up and look for the circumstances they want, and if they can't find them, make them."* — George Bernard Shaw[3]

A big reason why we struggle to move forward is because we are stuck in the past. Like I mentioned in the previous section, a lot of my clients struggled from what their parents ingrained in their minds as kids. They found it difficult to move forward towards positivity because they felt so terrible about themselves and had created a really negative perspective around who they were. While you are completely valid for feeling the way, you do about a certain aspect in your life, you also have to recognize that we need to move past the things we've experienced and not let them affect us now the way they did when we first felt them. What happened to you throughout your life that might have led to trauma and even PTSD is awful, and it hurts to think that so many people like me have suffered. However, we have to look at what happened and find a use for it now. The experiences we had, especially the tough ones, have only made us stronger and helped to build the amazing character that we have today.

It can also be hard to keep going because we can become so fearful of the future. When we experienced so much pain in the past, we start to think this is our reality, especially if we were children when we experienced the hard things, then we'll think that this is how the world works. It will be harder to move forward towards a positive experience when all we know is negativity and struggle. You have to make sure that you are doing your best to not let the things that happened to you define what you think about the future. Do not fear what we do not know.

The things that we experienced in our past, how we were raised, where we grew up, the mentality of our family members, and everything else that helped create who we are plays a huge role in your eating disorders now, there's no doubt about that. If you grew up in a fit household where healthy eating was encouraged but not enforced, then you probably have a good perspective on eating right. If you grew up where fast food was every other meal, and neither parent had the time to cook, then you're going to be a lot unhealthier.

The only thing you can do is focus on what is going on right now. You can't change the past and what happened to you, and we don't have the option of looking to the future to see what to expect. The only thing you have power over now is what's going on around you. If we don't focus on things that surround us at the moment, then we will quickly start to lose sight of reality, and the little time we have left will slip through our hands.

You can't change the past. You can affect the future, but you can never predict what's actually going to happen. The sooner we accept that, the easier it will be to move forward. If you want to learn more about overcoming your childhood trauma and looking at the past to see what might have caused your unhealthy mentality now, then I suggest making sure to check out the first book.

Those That Bring You Down

"Growing apart doesn't change the fact that for a long time we grew side by side; our roots will always be tangled. I'm glad for that." — Ally Condie[4]

Unfortunately, even our closest friends and family members can be the people that will bring us down. When I was going on through my weight loss journey, there were some friends that had been around my all my life that still weren't very supportive. This was hard to deal with. On one hand, I wanted to help make them less bitter, but on the other, I needed to focus on helping myself. Though I might have been friends with someone for a few years, if they weren't helping me in my journey and only adding negativity, then it wasn't helpful to keep them around. Sometimes you have to let someone go, and remove them from your life. If they aren't there to support and help you, remember that this is never your fault. Sometimes we simply grow apart from people.

Many women struggle with weight loss, especially because of the images and ideas put in their heads about body image by their mothers. This was very common when I would speak to a lot of my patients. They would either have mothers that belittled them for their bodies, or they had mothers that put themselves down, causing that mentality to form in their daughters. If you want to improve your health, that might include improving a relationship, especially with your mother.

People are going to try to discourage you, make you feel dumb, and judge what you are doing. Anyone that goes out of their way to make you feel bad has some serious problems of their own.

You can help certain people. Some individuals might be hurtful to you because they are jealous, resentful, or simply unhappy themselves. If you can encourage others to be healthier, inviting them out for a workout class or telling them how great they look on a regular basis. However, you can only help these people so much. If the other person isn't willing or wanting to change, we can't force them, and it's not our place to tell them that they need to change.

Be honest with what you are feeling and never feel ashamed to share that someone has hurt you. I noticed a lot of people saying things like, "you look so much better now!" after I had lost 90 pounds. I hated that. I knew I looked good and I loved that people could see how healthy I was, but I didn't want them to tell me I was better than I was before. I was still that girl that had the 90 pounds of extra weight on her, and I hated being compared by other people. When they said this, they were basically stating that I was prettier or more attractive since I had lost the weight. What would have been more helpful was if they had said things like, "you look so healthy now," "I can see how happy you are," or "it's great to see that you're feeling good about yourself." This was the goal of my weight loss journey, not just to get approval from others based on my level of attractiveness. I would call these people out and let them know that what they said was hurtful and that they should be careful with their words. Most people didn't realize what they were saying, but they should have, and it's important that we remind others to be mindful of the things they choose to say to us.

Remember that change lies within yourself, so some people just simply will be stuck in their ways as they navigate throughout life. It can be hard, but if you need to let someone go for the sake of your own mental health, then that's just the way it has to be.

Don't Be Self-Conscious at the Gym

A big struggle I had with my weight loss journey was the fear over what people would think of me as I walked down the street or worked out in the gym. I would avoid runs and never got a gym membership until a little way through my journey because I loathed what other people would say about me or my body. If only I would have known how unhealthy this mentality was, I would have lost the weight a lot sooner. Don't allow yourself to stop from doing something healthy just because you're afraid of what other people are going to think or say.

Everyone at the gym even the most fit guy of all, is going to be more focused on their own body than they will themselves. That's why there are so many mirrors at the gym, so people can look at themselves and the form that they have when they're lifting weights. People aren't going to look at you and think something bad, they'll more likely look at you and wonder if you are judging them!

If someone does judge you, stare too much, or even makes fun of you, then that's on them. You might run into the occasional bad seed in the gym, a person that laughs, mocks or rolls their eyes at you. I had a few people make smaller passive aggressive comments to me but letting that get to me never helped. Instead, I had to realize that I don't care about the opinions of people that so harshly judge others. Why would you ever judge someone so harshly for trying to lose weight? Why would you mock someone because they are struggling with their body image? A person like that isn't worth your time, especially time that you might skip out on at the gym.

You are not at fault for someone else's perceptions of you if they are a stranger. They might think terrible things about you. Everyone at the gym could even be judging you, you never know, you can't read minds. However, we can't let ourselves think this way! It's only going to hold us back. We have to remind ourselves of that, and the fact that if this were true, if they all were judging us, then who cares! They're the ones with the issues, not us. Never let the thought of other people hold you back.

Prove everyone wrong and show them that you aren't someone that should be judged. Keep going to the gym and focus on yourself. The more you remember this, the easier it will be for you to overcome any fear of working out in public.

1) Shakespeare, W., & Rollins, H. (1940). The passionate pilgrim.
2) Mure PhD, N. (2015.) EAT! Empower Adjust Triumph!
3) Shaw, B. (2017). Mrs. Warren's profession.
4) Condie, A., & Condie, A. (2010). Matched.

Chapter 7 - An Individual's Worth

"Am I less of a person because I weigh more?"
— Carol Riggs[1]

You are worth it! You have value! As someone overweight who struggled with body image, I know that this is the hardest thing to convince yourself. Saying no to the extra brownie or telling yourself that you can't skip another workout is hard. Reminding ourselves that we need to take care of who we are and keep moving forward is a challenge. However, the thing that is hardest out of all of that is telling ourselves that we are worth it. I told myself for so long that I wasn't, that I took up too much space and that I was a bad person for eating so much and never working out. However, this kind of mentality is what kept me so unmotivated for so long! As soon as I realized I was a person that deserved absolute greatness, I started to feel so much better about myself.

It is not selfish to take care of yourself! It makes you stronger to care for those you love! If you don't have love for yourself, where do you expect to get the love required to give to other people? I'm not going to lie; my weight affected my marriage for a bit. I didn't want to be affectionate because it felt unnatural. I spent so much time hating myself and breaking down who I was as a person that it started to leak into the way that I treated other people. When I started to really love the person that I was, it made it so much easier to share that love with other individuals.

It improves your moods and makes you more happy, positive and loving because you feel better, stronger and have more to give! When I was feeling low about myself and lacking self-confidence, I often questioned my worth. I would think, "what value do I have? Why should anyone else listen to me, or love me?" This kind of thinking made me believe that I had nothing to offer other people. Once I started to grow the compassion I had for myself and share that love with other individuals, it became easier to see my value. When I recognized my value, I could more easily share that with another pope because I believed in myself. I knew that I had something important inside of me that other people could benefit from, and that they wanted to listen to. When you can really learn how to love yourself and get to a point in your journey where you enjoy who you are and what you have become, then it teaches those around you to do the same. The thing that makes me a great parent is that I know I am a good person, and my sons can see that. Not only that, but they will also see their own value, making them stronger people as well. When you love yourself and really see your worth, it makes you an amazing role model to your family and your community!

Write in your journal every day one or more things you are grateful for! Some days, I'm grateful that I have people that love me. I count my blessings and see that there is so much about me that makes me who I am. I am grateful that I have had experiences that taught me about myself and I'm appreciative of the challenges I've experienced because they made me a better person. I write down every day at least one thing I'm grateful for, but other days I'll write an entire entry. It might be something as simple as finding a cute top on the clearance rack, or something more serious like everyone coming out unharmed after a car accident. Whatever it is, write down and share with yourself the things that you are grateful for. Read it again before you start your day. You will be amazed how this simple act can put your mind in a healthy way!

The most successful thing we will be able to do is to be authentically ourselves. There are so many people that imitate others, copy their looks, and try to think in a certain way that aligns with the beliefs of others. Once we start to act like another person and lose who we really are, then we are no longer the same person. The best way to find the most success is to keep going through this life as your own.

Loving yourself is going to take you much farther than hating yourself ever did.

Weight Loss Affirmations

"Like all living things, you were created for unlimited growth and possibilities. Keep

growing. Keep changing. Be everything you were meant to be." — Eleanor Brownn[2]

Weight loss affirmations are phrases that will help you to overcome your doubts and fears and plant new ideas in your head. You need to surround yourself with weight loss affirmations. These include phrases including "I am," "I can," "I will," and so on. You should write them down in your journal put a poster of them on the wall by your treadmill and repeat them to yourself over and over again. The more we can share these weight loss affirmations with ourselves, the easier it will be to overcome all the challenges that we have to face.

We have repeatedly told ourselves things that have made it challenging to really find the success that we want. You have to start right now turning that energy around. Our minds will take on things simply because they have been exposed to them for so long. Think of a favorite teacher you had as a child. There was a good chance that they had a poster in their room that really affected you, or perhaps a phrase that stuck with you since then. This is because our minds pick up on that phrasing and then repeat it over and over again. The more you repeat something, the likelier it will be for you to accept this as the truth. That is why we need affirmations. They will be phrases that we can say to ourselves when we want to give up when we need motivation, and simply as a way to start our day. Even repeating, "I can do this," to myself over and over again as I walk to the gym or drive to the rec center can be enough for me to keep pushing forward.

Come up with your own affirmations. These are some great examples of weight loss affirmations that have helped me a ton:

- I am capable
- I am strong
- I am healthy
- I am doing this because I deserve to
- No one is in charge but me
- I love my body
- I am patient and am willing to work for results
- This will take time, and I am ready
- I am strong enough to push through the hardest parts
- I am passionate enough to do this and finish with success

You might also find success from using weight loss meditation. There are books on these as well as plenty of YouTube videos. Meditation is a great way for you to focus on yourself, your mind, and your body, and get to a place where you can easily relax and distress. While you meditate, you might try to listen to one specified towards weight loss or including affirmations that will help drive the idea that you deserve so much more in a more comprehensive manner.

Write to Yourself When in a Good Mood

We talked a lot about the importance of journaling. It is a way to help you organize your thoughts. Make sure that you are doing this just as often when you are in good moods as you are when you are feeling low or triggered. At first, I would only write in my journal when I was feeling down about myself. I would write entries on being sad and I would consistently think about how I needed to write about the hard times to get through them. Then, one day, I realized that I need to be writing in my journal every day, especially on the good days! When I do this, I connect all my thoughts together and have a place to go to where I can look at my thought process and better understand all the patterns of thinking that makeup who I am.

I have notes in my journals that say things like, "remember how good it feels to be this happy!" I don't instantly become happy, but it does remind me on my darkest days that this is not how life is every day. I'll write a letter about the good emotions I have, what that feels like, and what they might have been triggered by. The better I can create positivity in my journal, the easier it will be to remember this kind of emotion when I'm in a bad mood.

You will have your ups and downs. Our emotions can sometimes even be like a pendulum. The bigger the pendulum swings in one direction, the higher it will go in the other. If you are having a terrible mood one day, then you might have a seemingly perfect one the next. No matter what happens, you will need to focus on your emotional state and see how you might be peaking in one direction or the other to track your moods. Though we will always have ups and downs, if we are aware of our triggers and what goes into lower moods, then it will be easier to understand how to get out of a bad mood when one comes along. Hopefully, we get to a place where there are more good moods than bad, but we have to be realistic.

When you journal when you are happy, it gives you the perspective needed to make it through the tough times. Since you should be your own best friend, this means also including advice on how to improve moods and reminders that you will get through it. Write letters to yourself when you're in a good mood. I have a letter to myself for when I'm feeling self-conscious, angry about my past, and wanting to quit altogether. When I'm in that mood, I can go to that specific letter and read it from my own words, in my own voice, with my own thought patterns. This helps remind me that the bad mood is just a temporary feeling that I've had before, with the letters as proof that I've managed to make it out at one point before at the very least.

Mental Fitness

Your mental fitness is going to be just as important as your physical fitness. Workout your brain like you would your muscles. Make sure that you are focusing on improving your thinking patterns and all of the negative thoughts that might go into who you are as a person. It is going to take time to see improvement, especially with your positive thoughts. It can be very easy to fall into one kind of thinking. Remind yourself that nothing is off limits. And the things that you are already thinking aren't always concrete or necessarily true either.

Rework Your Relationship with Food

"It involved giving up what I thought was bringing me comfort, only to clearly see they were leading to a sure and certain early death. I was committing suicide slowly, sweet morsel by sweet morsel." — Teresa Shields Parker[3]

The reason why dieting can be so hard is because of the way that we interact with food. For some people, it is a comforting aspect, and other people are afraid of food because of how much power it has over them. Unfortunately, we can't just quit eating. If you were an alcoholic, you could give up beer, wine, and liquor, and never step foot in a bar again. Unfortunately, we have to eat to survive. There's no getting rid of our need to eat, so we have to figure out how to create a healthy relationship with the foods that we decide to eat.

Let it be an experience, not just something that you put in your mouth. Don't eat in front of the TV anymore. I would eat dinner a lot while watching TV,

157

and then I would simply stuff my face without really thinking about it. What would end up happening was that I was binge eating and going way past my limit. When I could sit down at a table and talk to my family while eating, I was much more likely to control the amount and far less likely to be binge eating. We have to be mindful with the things we decide to eat.

One thing that helps me is to cook dinner for other people, especially my family. I like making food that other people like and making them happy by sharing not only tasty dishes but healthy ones too. It feels good to accomplish something, and other people telling me they like my food or that I'm a good cook helps me to build my confidence.

Break up with the foods that you are already eating. It can be easy to fall into a pattern of comfortable eating. I would eat chips all the time, all night and throughout the day. I realized one day that I didn't even like chips that much. I would just sit there and repeatedly eat these things just because I was bored and wanted something to do with my hands. I stopped buying chips and instead started doing other things to take up my time, like doing crossword puzzles and even knitting. I never thought about chips anymore and instead just focused on what my next project would be.

Start Cooking

Cooking is the best way for me to connect back to my food. It gives you control over the things that you eat so you can make sure no sneaky foods are making their way into your body.

It has become therapeutic for me. I also love experimenting. I enjoy buying weird food and seeing what dish I can make. It has helped my family become healthier and more adventurous eaters as well. I use fresh herbs to season my dishes and am always excited when the grocery store features a produce item that I haven't used before. I sometimes even like to imagine I'm on a cooking show that challenges me to use a difficult ingredient.

If you hate cooking, ask yourself why? For a while, I disliked it because I didn't know how. I would burn eggs and somehow even my spaghetti tasted strange. However, I realized that cooking is simply something that we have to practice. You're not going to be a master chef overnight, but the more effort you put into improving, the better you will be in the end.

Once you start to grocery shop for mindfulness and prepare your own meals, it will start to decrease your desire to go out. I realized now that when I go to certain restaurants, I think of how I might have been able to make that dish better! I don't share this because I don't want to make anyone feel bad about themselves, but there are some dishes where you can tell not as much effort. Was put in. it makes me want to stay home and cook for myself instead because I know I have what it takes to make it tasty for myself.

1) Riggs, C. (2015). The Body Institute.
2) Brownn, E. (2009). Mile 9: The true story of a lifelong couch potato who one day made a decision that changed everything.
3) Parker, T. (2013). Sweet Grace: How I Lost 250 Pounds and Stopped Trying to Earn God's Favor.

Chapter 8 - Live in Gratitude

"Be grateful for what you already have while you pursue your goals. If you aren't grateful for what you already have, what makes you think you would be happy with more." — Roy T. Bennett[1]

It can be easy to feel bad about ourselves and our health. There are so many people out there that are struggling with things they have no control over – cancer, diseases, physical handicaps. Be grateful that you've struggled with your weight. It is given you such an amazing perspective.

Greatness already exists, we just have to find it. When you exude confidence and happiness, it can be contagious. It will be easier each and every day to be positive the more and more we practice.

"However, mean your life is, meet it and live it; do not shun it and call it hard names. It is not so bad as you are. It looks poorest when you are richest. The fault-finder will find faults even in paradise. Love your life, poor as it is. You may perhaps have some pleasant, thrilling, glorious hours, even in a poorhouse. The setting sun is reflected from the windows of the almshouse as brightly as from the rich man's abode; the snow melts before its door as early in the spring. I do not see but a quiet mind may live as contentedly there, and have

as cheering thoughts, as in a palace." —
Henry David Thoreau[2]

Help Others Achieve What You Have Achieved

You should start a blog or at least share with friends on social media what contributed to your success so they can become inspired! Send a "thinking of you" card to a dieting coworker telling her that you can tell she is losing weight, that you believe in her and you admire her tenacity!

Donate your nice clothes that are too big to a friend who is losing down herself and needs some new clothes! Share your weight loss success story with a local dieting support group. Giving back inspires you to stay on course for the long haul!

Having Fun with Exercise

Exercise was always a trigger for me. It is hard work! If it were easy, we would all be walking around with muscles ripping through our t-shirts. Find ways that exercise is fun. Dancing and going for walks are types of exercise that doesn't have to be strenuous. Buying workout clothes can really help too. Friends will make it easier. I avoided working out with others for a while because I was scared of them judging me.

Diet Mentality

"Every weight loss program, no matter how positively it is packaged, whispers to you that you are not right. You are not good enough. You are unacceptable and you need to be fixed." — Kim Brittingham[3]

We have to address the "diet" mentality that many people have. In our society, where billions of dollars go into workout gear and other fitness products, it's important to understand how toxic this kind of thinking can be.

Monday was always a day for me to start my diet. If I failed, I kept thinking, "next week," as if something magical was going to come along that helped me to lose weight. Looking great is just a side effect, not something that you should focus on.

Years ago, it was actually a positive to be overweight because it showed that you had wealth. In the early 2000s, low-rise jeans were popular, and those only looked good on people with extremely flat stomachs. Trends will always come and go, so you have to remember that it should never be about the way that you look, but how you are feeling. What matters more than anything is that you are healthy and taking care of yourself.

"Here's the truth of the matter: It is not your fault that you don't already have the body you

want. It is the weight loss industry's fault." —
Mason Harder[4]

1) Bennett, R. (2016). <u>The Light in the Heart.</u>
2) Brittingham, K. (2011). <u>Read my hips.</u>
3) Harder, M. (2018). <u>The Phentermine & Clenbuterol Sourcebook: Cycling Weight Loss Pills to Burn Fat Fast, the Keto Diet on Steroids.</u>

Conclusion

If you are losing weight and going through this journey, then you are taking care of yourself, and that means that you are taking care of yourself mentally as well. Deciding that you need a change is going to be the first sign of self-love. Do this because you want to take care of yourself, not just because you want to punish yourself. When you realize that you need to do this for health and happiness, it will be a lot easier to keep moving in a direction of positive change.

Perfection is so boring. The most interesting things come from what separates us and the struggles that we have gone through. There are people who seem perfect that we admire, but do you really want to be friends with them? To me, being with someone that was perfect and has no flaws sounds scary, and honestly, kind of boring. Our loved ones are our best friends because they are flawed. They are funny, they are silly, they say strange things, and they do weird things. We relate to each other based on our similar thought patterns and we enjoy the interest that our differences bring. They are flawed, have made mistakes, and will still have moments that they mess up in the future. But we love them, and to us, they are perfect.

This is how we need to start seeing ourselves.

Thank you!

Thank you so much for reading my book!

I hope that you enjoyed the experience. I truly wanted you to obtain what you need to care for yourself and to regain and/or maintain your health!

Please remember that independent authors live and die (professionally) by the reviews that are left for us.

Please be so kind as to leave a review on Amazon after reading my book.

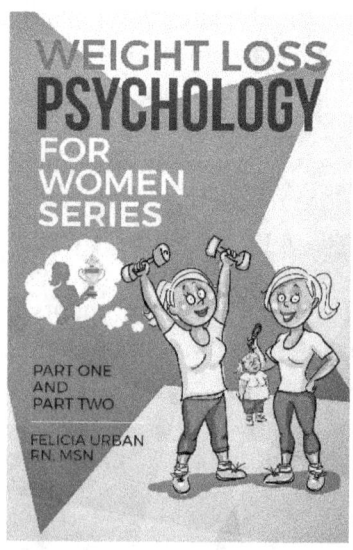

Interested in more content by
Felicia Urban?

Come visit us on the Weight Loss Psychology
Series website and don't forget to hit that
subscribe button to stay up to date on all new
content! https://geni.us/WLPSeries

Interact with Weight Loss Psychology community
by joining the Facebook page

Interact with Weight Loss Psychology community
by joining the Facebook group

Interested in the author and her other books?
Take a look on Amazon

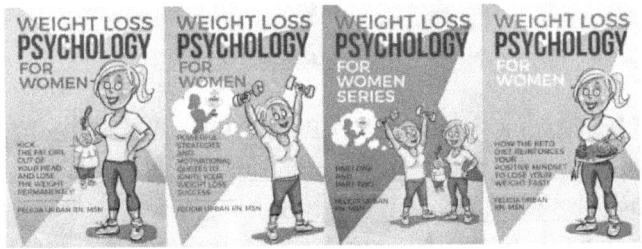

References

Bennett, R. (2016). The Light in the Heart.

Berkhan, M. (2018). The Leangains Method.

Bond, H. (2015). Who's the new kid?

Brittingham, K. (2011). Read my hips.

Brownn, E. (2009). Mile 9: The true story of a lifelong couch potato who one day made a decision that changed everything.

Condie, A., & Condie, A. (2010). Matched.

Confucius., & Waley, A. (2000). The Analects.

Cunningham, T., & Skolnik, H. (2010). The Reverse Diet.

Deuty, S. (2019). Secrets of an Over 50 Former Fat Man.

Frankl, V. (1946). Man's search for meaning.

Harder, M. (2018). The Phentermine & Clenbuterol Sourcebook: Cycling Weight Loss Pills to Burn Fat Fast, the Keto Diet on Steroids.

Kalantri, A. (2019). Wealth of Words.

Maraboli, S. (2014). Life, the truth, & being free.

Murayama, K. (2019). The science of motivation.

Mure PhD, N. (2015). EAT! Empower Adjust Triumph!

Parker, T. (2013). Sweet Grace: How I Lost 250 Pounds and Stopped Trying to Earn God's Favor.

Riggs, C. (2015). The Body Institute.

Roosevelt, E. (2018). Autobiography of Eleanor Roosevelt.

Shakespeare, W., & Rollins, H. (1940). The passionate pilgrim.

Shaw, B. (2017). Mrs. Warren's profession.

Society for Personality and Social Psychology. (2014). How we form habits, change existing ones.

Sorenson, T. (2019). The Great Brain Cleanse.

Spangle, L. (2007). 100 Days of Weight Loss: The Secret to Spangle, L.

WEIL, S. (2018). Changeability.

Ziglar, Z. (2010). Raising positive kids in a negative world.